COW TALK

UNDERSTANDING DAIRY COW BEHAVIOUR
TO IMPROVE THEIR WELFARE ON ASIAN FARMS

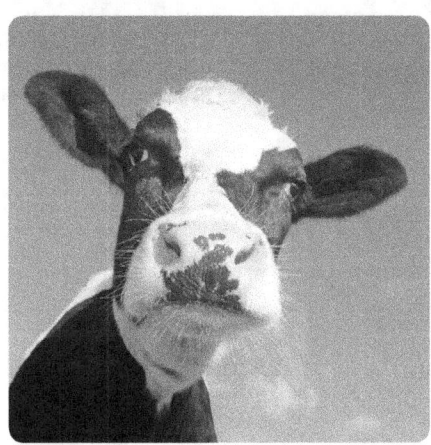

JOHN MORAN AND REBECCA DOYLE

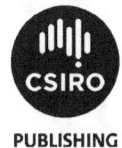

CSIRO

PUBLISHING

National Library of Australia Cataloguing-in-Publication entry

> Moran, John, 1945– author.
> Cow talk : understanding dairy cow behaviour to improve their welfare on Asian farms / John Moran and Rebecca Doyle.
> 9781486301614 (paperback)
> 9781486301621 (epdf)
> 9781486301638 (epub)
>
> Includes bibliographical references and index.
> Dairy cattle – Behavior.
> Cattle – Behavior.
> Cows – Behavior.
> Animal welfare – Asia.
>
> Doyle, Rebecca, author.
>
> 636.44095

Published by

CSIRO Publishing
36 Gardiner Road, Clayton VIC 3168
Private Bag 10, Clayton South VIC 3169
Australia

Telephone: [+613] 9545 8555
Email: csiropublishing@csiro.au
Website: www.publishing.csiro.au

All photographs are by John Moran unless otherwise indicated

Front cover: Sebastian Knight/Shutterstock.com

Set in 11/13.5 Minion & Helvetica Neue
Edited by Anne Findlay, Editing Works Pty Ltd
Cover design by James Kelly
Typeset by Thomson Digital
Printed by Ingram Lightning Source

CSIRO Publishing publishes and distributes scientific, technical and health science books and journals from Australia to a worldwide audience and conducts these activities autonomously from the research activities of the Commonwealth Scientific and Industrial Research Organisation (CSIRO). The views expressed in this publication are those of the author(s) and do not necessarily represent those of, and should not be attributed to, the publisher or CSIRO. The copyright owner shall not be liable for technical or other errors or omissions contained herein. The reader/user accepts all risks and responsibility for losses, damages, costs and other consequences resulting directly or indirectly from using this information.

Foreword

How many academic books lie languishing on library shelves, a tribute to the authors, but of little practical value? Not this one! This book will fulfil a vital role in disseminating research findings to those directly involved in cow husbandry – farmers, vets, agricultural advisers and students. Available to be freely downloaded, this book goes a long way towards filling that major void between the researchers in dairy cow management and those actually doing the work with the cows. And all this was generously made possible by the Crawford Foundation, providing the necessary funds so that the publishers can offer the book free of charge.

The authors, John Moran and Rebecca Doyle, have both been intimately involved in livestock management. Their role in this book, as in John's four previous tropical dairy management books, is to take major texts on the topic and distil them into something that can be used by those working with cows, herdspersons, vets etc. John has spent several decades consulting to the dairy industry, both in Australia and SE Asia and has produced many books, CDs, trainee manuals and journal articles with a dairy extension focus. Rebecca has recently been appointed as a Research Fellow at the Animal Welfare Science Centre at the University of Melbourne and has specialised in livestock emotions for her PhD and subsequent research work.

The book starts with the premise that demand for dairy produce is growing, particularly in Asia where inhabitants are, rightly or wrongly, changing to a Western diet. Unfortunately keeping dairy cows in tropical conditions in developing countries is fraught with risks to their welfare, and performance is usually well below that achieved in Western countries. Although many Asian developing countries are currently importing much of their requirements from the West, most governments there have the intention to expand and develop efficient dairy industries, in which the cows' needs are adequately met.

The book lays the foundation for a sound understanding of how to look after cows by first describing their senses in some detail. The authors tell us how cows talk to each other and how they talk to us, although we often ignore this. Moving into welfare management, the authors describe the signals that cattle provide when their welfare is compromised, from the more obvious ones such as body posture and condition to the more subtle ones, such as rumination and eye white area. Yes, cows' eyelids open wider when they are startled just like ours, revealing more eye white. Who would have thought of looking for the 'presence of cobwebs in the cowshed (because it) is indicative of low air movement'. Scoring systems are presented that are practical and help novices in particular to describe key features of cow welfare, such as body condition, feet, cleanliness and lameness. Documenting what we see helps us to both remember and compare. As research tools, they must be used judiciously.

Much is written about good handling techniques, because poor handling is at the root of many welfare problems for dairy cows. Having an empathetic, experienced and knowledgeable herdsperson is the key to minimising handling risks, or should it be a cowperson? The authors coin a new term, cowpersonship, which emphasises the importance for every person of understanding each cow, rather than just the herd. Many books fall into the trap of prescribing conditions for the average cows, whereas this book focuses on variation between individual cows and the importance of providing for the welfare of all. Hence the need for good cow observation skills, not easy when intensification is resulting in less and less time being available to spend with the cows. It is no coincidence that in intensive cow units it is getting harder to repeatedly get the cows pregnant, which requires the cowperson to observe oestrous behaviour in a cow if he or she wants to artificially inseminate her. Another meaningful term then emerges, namely, farm blindness (or being unable to see when something is wrong on a farm). Despite the authors' recognition of the essentiality of good cowpersonship, they acknowledge that skilled workers are increasingly hard to find, particularly in situations in which there are competing industries offering higher salaries and better working conditions.

The authors caution of the dangers in going down the route of intensification, using cows that are genetically predisposed to give large quantities of milk, as it often leads to poor welfare and performance. In their words, 'we breed cows to produce more and more milk at the expense of their welfare'. Intensive housing is also critically reviewed for all its faults in attending to cows' daily needs, potentially leading to behaviour problems such as aggression, kicking, and stereotyped tongue rolling. Keeping cows indoors in tie stalls is common in SE Asia due to the shortage of land for grazing systems. Too many potentially high yielding dairy cows have been sent from Australia and New Zealand to SE Asia, only for farmers to find that the cows lose condition and have an appetite that is almost impossible to satisfy, with the result that the milk yields are low and the cows barren. Heat stress compounds this welfare insult.

This book takes a lot of the dairy cow research material that has been generated in the last 20 years and interprets it for the farmer, extracting what is useful in the work that has been done. It is not a lengthy academic text that is entirely evidence-based and copiously referenced, but it is eminently suitable for practising farmers, students and academics who are looking for practical information on cow management. Much of what is written appears common sense and easily put into practice, until you realise the commercial pressures that many in the dairy industry have to submit to.

The book concludes with the advice that 'Happy cows make happy farmers'. I'd guarantee that all dairy farmers will find something in this book that helps to make their cows, and them, just that little bit happier.

Clive Phillips
Centre for Animal Welfare and Ethics
University of Queensland, Gatton, Australia
Email: c.phillips@uq.edu.au

Contents

About the authors

John Moran

For 30 years, Dr John Moran was an Australian senior research and advisory scientist from Victoria's Department of Primary Industries (DPIV), located in northern Victoria. Over the last 10 years he spent half his time advising farmers in southern Australia and half his time working with dairy farmers and advisers in South and East Asia. His specialist fields include dairy production, ruminant nutrition, calf and heifer rearing, forage conservation and whole farm business management. Following his retirement from DPIV in June 2011, John formed a consulting business, Profitable Dairy Systems, located in Kyabram.

John graduated in 1967 with a Rural Science honours degree from New England University at Armidale in NSW, followed by a Masters degree in 1969. In 1976, he obtained a Doctorate of Philosophy in beef production from University of London, Wye College in England. During the 1980s, John lived in Indonesia for 3 years, working in beef cattle and buffalo research. Since 1999, he initiated and conducted training programs on smallholder dairy production to farmers, advisers and policy makers in Indonesia, Malaysia, Thailand, Vietnam, China, Pakistan, Sri Lanka, Bangladesh, Myanmar and East Timor. In 2013 he was appointed as Coordinator of the Asia Dairy Network, an international agency position to facilitate communication and collaboration of dairy industries from 15 countries throughout South and East Asia.

As a result of his Asian programs, in 2005 John wrote his first dairy manual, *Tropical Dairy Farming: Feeding Management for Small Holder Dairy Farmers in the Humid Tropics*. As well as hard copy, the book was published on the internet, making it freely available to dairy stakeholders throughout the world. In 2008 John wrote his second manual on tropical dairy farming, namely *Business Management for Tropical Dairy Farmers*. By August 2014, these two books had received over 250 000 'hits' on the internet, indicating their relevance particularly to Asian tertiary teaching institutes and government livestock departments.

The indepth review he conducted during a LIVECORP consultancy on developing management packages for tropical dairy production technology formed the basis of his third book, entitled *Managing High Grade Dairy Cows in the Tropics*. His fourth book, entitled *Rearing Young Stock on Tropical Dairy Farms in Asia,* was an update of one of his earlier books, but written specifically for tropical smallholder farmers. This, his fifth book on tropical dairy farming, concentrates on animal welfare, a very valid topic for the current emphasis on the importation of exotic dairy heifers to many tropical countries.

John has published more than 200 research papers and advisory articles. He has also written several farmer manuals on dairy and beef cattle nutrition, veal production calf and heifer rearing and on silage production. The first edition of *Calf Rearing: A Guide to Rearing Calves in Australia*, published in 1993, sold more than 10 000 copies. The second edition, published in 2002, is still selling widely throughout Australia. He also published a companion book on young stock management, *Heifer Rearing: A Guide to Rearing Dairy Replacement Heifers in Australia*. His book, *Forage Conservation: Making Quality Silage and Hay in Australia*, published in 1996, is now a set text for undergraduate study in several Australian universities. One of his latest books, *Feedpads for Grazing Dairy Cows*, which he wrote in 2010 with his DPI colleague Scott McDonald, is also a bestseller in the dairy industry. All books are commercially available through CSIRO Publications on <http://www.publish/csiro/au>.

John's initial training in a systems approach to livestock science, together with his many years working closely with dairy industries in Australia and South and East Asia stand him in great stead to write this fifth tropical manual, *Cow Talk: Understanding Dairy Cow Behaviour to Improve Their Welfare on Asian Farms* which complements his previous books.

Rebecca Doyle

As an early career researcher, Rebecca has worked in the area of ruminant welfare since 2007, commencing with a PhD on sheep behaviour with CSIRO and the University of New England. After completing her PhD in 2010, Rebecca joined Charles Sturt University in Wagga Wagga, NSW as lecturer in animal physiology and welfare. She has recently been appointed as a Research Fellow at the Animal Welfare Science Centre in the University of Melbourne. She has worked with the beef cattle industry, both in Australia and Indonesia, to improve the welfare of exported cattle. In addition, Rebecca has conducted stock handling and welfare training programs for export sheep in the Middle East. With her experience in cattle behaviour and welfare, she has contributed to several chapters in this book.

Other books and technical manuals written by the senior author

Books

Calf Rearing: A Guide to Rearing Calves in Australia (1993)

Forage Conservation: Making Quality Silage and Hay in Australia (1996)

Heifer Rearing: A Guide to Rearing Dairy Replacement Heifers in Australia (with Douglas McLean) (2001)

Calf Rearing: A Practical Guide (2002)

Tropical Dairy Farming: Feeding Management for Small Holder Dairy Farmers in the Humid Tropics (2005)

Business Management for Tropical Dairy Farmers (2009)

Feedpads for Grazing Dairy Cows (with Scott McDonald) (2010)

Fifty Years of Farmer Extension for Victoria's Dairy Industry (2011)

Managing High Grade Dairy Cows in the Tropics (2012)

Rearing Young Stock on Tropical Dairy Farms in Asia (2012)

Feeding Management of Small Holder Dairy Cattle and Buffalo in Tropical Asia: An E-Learning Course (2013)

Technical manuals

Maize for Fodder: A Guide to Growing, Conserving and Feeding Irrigated Maize in Northern Victoria (with Ken Pritchard) (1987)

Growing Calves for Pink Veal: A Guide to Rearing, Feeding and Managing Calves for Pink Veal in Australia (1990)

Growing Quality Forages for Small Holder Dairy Farms in Indonesia (2001)

Managing Dairy Farm Costs: Strategies for Dairy Farmers in Irrigated Northern Victoria (2002)

Feeding Management for Small Holder Dairy Farmers in Thailand (2002)

Improving Milk Composition through Better Feeding Management (2003)

The Key Drivers of Good Reproductive Performance on Indonesian Dairy Farms (2006)

Value Adding Indonesia's Dairy Industry: Developing Cottage Industries in East Java (2006)

Improving Business Skills of Small Holder Dairy Farmers in Thailand (2007)

Dairy Production in Malaysia with Particular Reference to Milk Quality (2007)

Dairy Production in Indonesia with Particular Reference to Milk Quality (2007)
Developing a Post-Arrival Herd Management Protocol for Imported Australian Dairy Heifers (2007)
Managing Heat Stress and Housing for Pakistani Dairy Cows and Buffaloes (2007)
Dairy Production from Small Holder Farmers in Asia: Synopses of Workshops from 2000 to 2007 (2008)
Dairy Production in Sri Lanka: Current Situation and Future Prospects (2008)
Improving Business Skills in Vietnam's Small Holder Dairy Industry (2008)
A Guide to Better Dairy Herd Management in the Tropics (2009)
Best Management Practices for Small Holder Dairy Farmers in Asia (2010)
Developing a Blueprint for a 50 Cow Small Holder Dairy Farm in Asia (2010)
The Nutritive Value of Feedstuffs for Dairy Farmers in South-East Asia (2012)
A Blueprint for a Large-Scale Intensive Dairy Farm in Asia (2012)
Developing Standard Operating Procedures for the Welfare of Australian Dairy Heifers in Overseas Markets (2013)
The Feeding of By-Products on Small Holder Dairy Farms in Asia and Other Tropical Regions (2014)
The Development and Self-Sufficiencies of Asia's Dairy Industries (2014)

Acknowledgements

We would like to gratefully acknowledge the CSIRO Publishing team, especially Ted Hamilton, who very professionally converted all our laptop computer writings to both a 'hard copy' book and a collection of PDF files.

As with John's first four books for Asian small holder dairy farmers, our gratitude also goes out to ATSE Crawford Fund, headed in Victoria by Ted Hayes, who provided generous financial support for this and all John's previous books. This support has allowed us to make this book freely available to anyone keen to better understand how dairy stock interact among themselves and with their 'keepers'.

The photograph standards in Chapter 6 were kindly provided by Ton van Schie, Publisher, Roodbont Agricultural Publishers, Zutphen, The Netherlands, from their published books *Cow Signals* and *Cow Signals Checkbook*, Vetvice/Roodbont Publishers B.V. (www.roodbont.com www.roodbont.nl).

Ms Kate Blaszak, of World Society for Protection of Animals, Sydney, provided relevant information from her studies of dairy cow welfare in Asian smallholder dairy farms.

Dr Jan Hulsen, of Vetvice, Bergen op Zoom, Netherland, provided us with valuable insights in cow behaviour, cow signals and how they relate to cow wellbeing. He was the author of the two key books on *Cow Signals*. Some of the pictures were supplied by:

Meat & Livestock Australia
Kate Blaszak
Philip Schultz
Denise Burrell
Roodbont Agricultural Publishers, Zutphen, Netherland
We are also grateful to our team of peer reviewers who provided their thoughts on how to make the book more readable to both technical and lay people readers.

Dr John Moran
Director, Profitable Dairy Systems, 24 Wilson St, Kyabram Victoria, 3620 Australia
Tel: +61 418 379 652 (mobile)
Email: jbm95@hotmail.com
Website: www.profitabledairysystems.com.au

Dr Rebecca Doyle
Research Fellow, Animal Welfare Science Centre, University of Melbourne,
Parkville, Victoria 3010, Australia
Tel: +61 3 9035 7535
Mobile: +61 417 419 501
Email: Rebecca.doyle@unimelb.edu.au
Website: www.animalwelfare.net.au

Acknowledgement of
The Crawford Fund

The publication of this book would not have been possible without the generous assistance of The Crawford Fund whose mission is to increase Australia's engagement in international agricultural research, development and education for the benefit of developing countries and Australia.

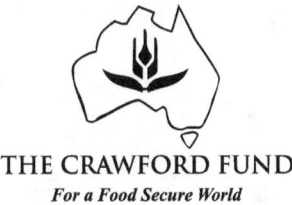

THE CRAWFORD FUND
For a Food Secure World

It is well demonstrated that educating handlers on animal welfare and behaviour has positive impacts on both the animals and workers. The aim of this book is to do just that.

Chemical warning

The registration and directions for use of chemicals can change over time. Before using a chemical or following any chemical recommendations, the user should ALWAYS check the uses prescribed on the label of the product to be used. If the product has not been recently produced, users should contact the place of purchase, or their local reseller, to check that the product and its uses are still registered. Users should note that the currently registered label should ALWAYS be used.

1

Introduction

This chapter presents an outline of the book. It highlights the importance of improved understanding of dairy cow behaviour and how this behaviour changes under small holder dairy (SHD) farm management.

The main points of this chapter

- In the process of developing tropical SHD farms, farmers and animal researchers have taken a domesticated species of livestock and greatly changed its physical and social environment.
- Animal welfare is important for producers because it can affect the health, production and contentment of cows. Having an understanding of factors that influence welfare can have important implications for production.
- South and East Asia are growing markets for imported dairy products as well as imported dairy stock to increase domestic milk production.
- Greater attention should be placed on management practices in tropical SHD farms to reduce any adverse effects on cow welfare and production.
- It can take up to 6 months for imported temperate dairy heifers to fully adapt to the living conditions of a tropical SHD farm.
- The wants and needs of dairy cows have been summarised as nine key factors.

1.1   What this book is all about

This book is primarily about how dairy (and beef) cattle communicate between themselves and with their keepers, namely the stockmen, women and farmers who run their everyday lives. Cattle are naturally gregarious animals preferring to socialise in groups, rather than as individuals. They also prefer space to congestion. Space allows them to sort out their social dominance relationships so the more subordinate cows can rest away from their dominant herd mates. When constricted in sheds, such social grouping is more difficult. Free stalls provide a sanctuary for submissive cows while the tie stall barn virtually removes such social interrelationships altogether.

The husbandry or management of cattle evolved many centuries ago in large areas of natural vegetation where the animals could freely graze. However, nowadays on most Asian farms livestock are restricted to small sheds where they are dependent on their keepers to supply them with everything from feed and water to minimised climate stresses and health support. Likewise, as a full range of natural behaviours when on heat cannot be expressed in small spaces or when tethered, stockpeople have had to be more adept at detecting cows on heat. This means that natural systems, where cows respond positively to the bull's attention, have had to be altered and now it is the person in charge of stock who identify signs of heat, then seek the bull or source the semen for artificial insemination.

The high cost of land, due to population pressures, and the low cost of labour, arising from the socioeconomic factors in developing countries, have led to continual shedding of stock. Even in developed countries, the more intensively managed cattle are housed. However, where possible, cattle are run outdoors because of the high costs of sourcing feed and water and the capital costs of infrastructure. Labour inputs are grossly different, for example, one stockperson can manage over 100 grazing dairy cows in Australia in contrast to only 20 fully housed cows in Asia.

When stock are housed in the tropics, sheds need to be designed and built to optimise natural ventilation and provide a flooring that is easy to clean yet comfortable to walk and rest on. High roofs and open sides together with gently sloping cement floors and specific cow resting areas on bedding material or mats are common features in well-designed sheds. The resting area should provide stock with non-abrasive bedding materials as well as a comfortable place and space to relax so they are able to more efficiently generate more of the products for which they are farmed, namely milk, meat and calves. Enduring climatic stresses such as high temperature and humidity are generally easier to cope with in the open, provided shade is available and access to natural ventilation is not impaired. It requires careful planning in a cowshed.

By concentrating stock in small or highly stocked areas, not only is it less natural for the stock to exhibit their normal behaviour, but it also provides an ideal environment for the propagation of pathogens. Therefore, attention to stock hygiene and health management must be prioritised to ensure stock do not unduly suffer from the intensive stock diseases associated with hard cement floors, manure and high density housing, namely lameness, mastitis, infectious diseases and respiratory problems.

Housing also means complete dependence on their keepers for feed and water. Even when provided with free grazing, cows depend greatly on the ability of the farmer to provide a diet balanced for the essential nutrients of profitable livestock performance. Out in the field grazing stock can select the most palatable, and presumably the most nutritious, parts of the plant. This is less likely to occur with most housed stock unless they are provided with large excesses, which increase wastage and reduce feeding profits. Hand-fed stock are entirely dependent on their keeper's skills to provide sufficient quantities of diet ingredients which can supply adequate amounts of feed nutrients and fibre to optimise their performance. This then assumes first, that the farmer has the knowledge and skills to formulate such a diet and second, the ingredients are available and so can be sourced at realistic prices to generate feeding profits.

Housing means increased interaction between stock and humans. The temperament of cattle can vary from wild, hardly tamed beef stock (commonly bulls) to quiet, very tractable and easily managed dairy cows. Housing can magnify the aggressive behaviour traits as cattle are forced to interact more closely with each other and with humans. As with any interaction between living creatures, communication is the key. Humans have developed language skills as the essence of such interaction, although non-verbal communication still plays an important part. Cattle have learnt to communicate between themselves through all their five senses while humans mainly communicate with animals using their ears and eyes and voice.

Communication between animals and humans then forms the basis of expressing the degree of stock comfort; that is how animals are at ease with their environment. If they are not comfortable and clearly indicate this state, it is up to humans to modify the environment to improve the animal's degree of comfort (see Figures 1.1 and 1.2). Unless they are made more comfortable, their primary objective, namely to produce saleable livestock products, will be compromised. If this is grossly compromised and sales of animal products are greatly reduced, their welfare can often be put at further risk, which indicates the humans' obligations to look after such animals are not being fulfilled.

Briefly, farmers and animal breeders have taken a domesticated species of livestock and completely changed its physical and social environment, particularly in the case of the SHD farmer in tropical Asia. After breeding and selecting the animal for high levels of production of livestock products of economic value (whether milk, live weight gain and/or calves), people then expect them to function

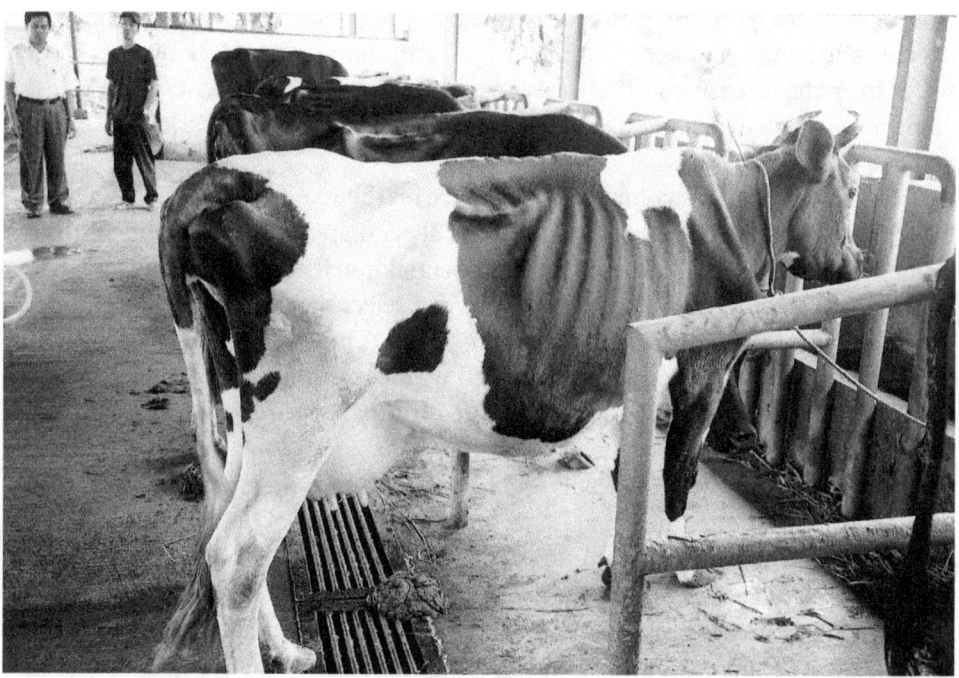

Figure 1.1: Very thin milking cows are an indicator of poor welfare, mainly due to poor feeding management.

in harmony with their new environment. It is only through better understanding and the provision of their needs to 'behave' normally, that we can hope to develop more profitable and sustainable systems of livestock farming. This then is the major objective of this book.

1.2   Outline of this book

This manual covers a wide range of topics primarily related to ensuring the sustainability of dairy production systems in tropical developing countries. Clearly, to achieve this aim, closer attention needs to be given to the economics of current systems. Sourcing high yielding dairy cows, but providing the feeding and management that only utilises a small proportion of their potential is just not sustainable in the long run. It is also a contributory factor to their suboptimal animal welfare because such animals are more susceptible to the traumas of heat stress, poor housing conditions and, all too often, subsistence feeding management.

This book is written for all the stakeholders in SHD production systems in the tropics, with an emphasis on South-East (SE) Asian countries. While small holders are the major suppliers of milk in the tropics, numerous larger farms are becoming established throughout the tropics to satisfy the increasing demands for fresh milk. It is hoped that both production systems farmers and their advisers will gain much

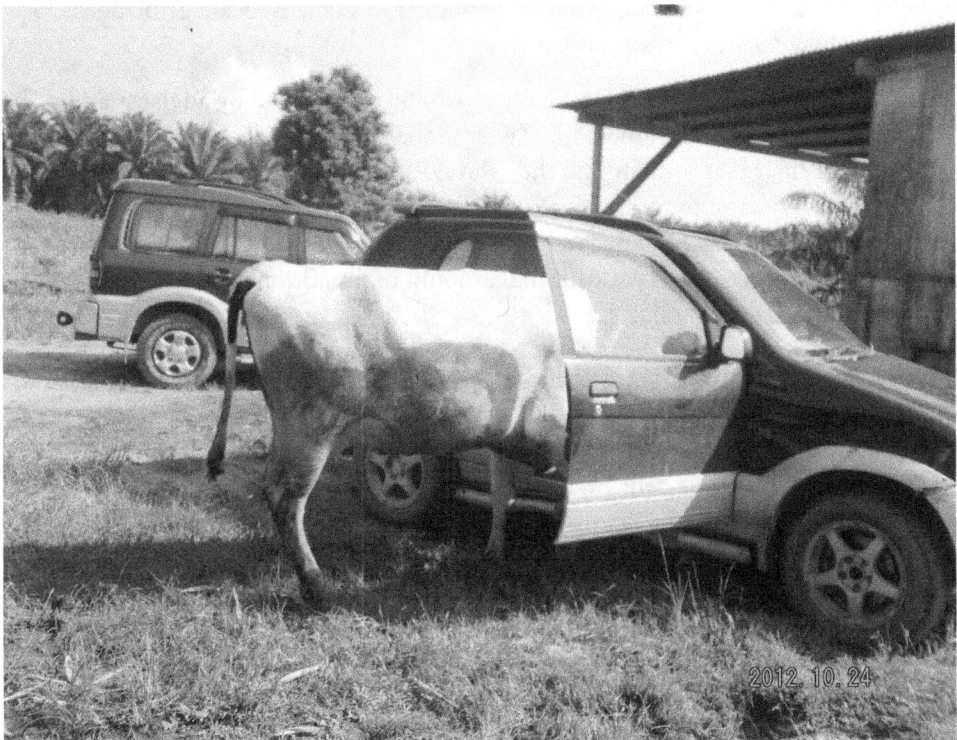

Figure 1.2: Cows are naturally curious creatures.

from this manual and improve the welfare and production of their cows. In addition, the book provides relevant key information from research scientists on aspects of cow behaviour and stock welfare. Policy makers and senior management should also benefit from reading selected chapters.

Most tropical countries have proactive programs to increase local supplies of milk, which require increasing numbers of well-trained workers to service their dairy industries. Consequently, educators from agricultural schools, universities and technical colleges need to be kept abreast of the latest technical developments and applications in dairy farming. This book also aims to serve this purpose.

The key target audiences for this book are:

- Farmers and stockpeople who want to improve and ensure adequate animal welfare.
- Farm advisers who can assist farmers to improve their welfare practices.
- Educators, usually at a technical level, who develop training programs for farmers.
- Educators, usually at a university level, who train dairy advisers in the basics of dairy production technology and stock welfare.

- Other stakeholders in tropical dairy production, such as local agribusiness, policy makers and research scientists.

These chapters are written so that they can be understood by advisers and tertiary students. As the trainers must ensure that other target audiences can comprehend their course material, they should select the most relevant sections to incorporate into basic programs for farmers. Each chapter has been written as a 'stand alone' document, which can be individually downloaded from the internet. For this reason, there may be a minimal amount of repetition between chapters. Chapter outlines are as follows:

- Chapter 2 provides an introduction to animal welfare, why it is important and the common welfare issues on dairy farms.
- Chapter 3 provides an insight into domestication, including the impact this has had on natural cattle behaviour.
- Chapter 4 discusses the details of cattle behaviour such as the five senses of the body, the various ways stock communicate with each other, behaviour indicating poor welfare, human–animal relationships and behavioural problems arising from clashes with their environment.
- Chapters 5 and 6 discuss practical signals you can use to assess cow wellbeing and welfare, how they can and should be interpreted and also how many of them have been quantified to improve the impact of their messages.
- Cow comfort is the topic of Chapter 7. This specifically covers what cow comfort is, the implications of this for welfare and how shed design and other facilities on the farm can influence this.
- Chapter 8 provides examples of farm audits and other ways to quantify animal welfare and its impact on dairy cow wellbeing and performance.
- Chapter 9 discusses the management of SE Asian SHD farms highlighting the key constraints to cow performance and how these impact on cow welfare.
- A protocol for the welfare of stock on tropical SHD farms is presented in Chapter 10.
- Chapter 11 concludes the manual with some final overviews.

Every profession has its jargon, or words developed specifically for that profession, and agriculture is no exception. There are some very specific terms and acronyms that are routinely used by dairy researchers and advisers. These are explained in the Glossary and when they are first mentioned in this manual. Full publication details of all sources of information are presented in the References and further reading section, while the Appendices include a list and websites of government and non-government agencies within Australia which are involved in cattle welfare. They also include checklists on how to quantify heat stress, what to look for when assessing good farm management and a simple scoring system of farm stock welfare. Finally, for ease of finding specific information, the Index lists all the key topics covered in the book and their relevant page numbers.

Many of the behavioural studies cited in this manual, particularly those in Chapters 3 and 4, have been reported in some of the standard textbooks on cattle behaviour, for example those written by Albright and Arave (1997), Grandin (1998), Phillips (2002) and Grandin (2007). As the actual researchers who conducted these studies were referenced by these textbook authors, they have not all been cited in this book. However, where a specific chapter has been written for an edited book, the original authors have been cited.

Several of the topics covered in this manual have previously been extensively reviewed in other books about tropical dairy farming, written by John Moran. Accordingly, duplication of these topics has been kept to a minimum by referring the reader to specific chapters in these previously published texts. All chapters of these books are freely downloadable on the Internet from the website <www.profitabledairysystems.com.au>. The full web addresses to source these books and chapters are also included in the bibliography of this book. Topics covered in specific chapters of previous texts include:

- Development of SHD farming in Asia; Chapter 3 of Moran (2009a)
- Body condition scoring; Chapter 18 of Moran (2005)
- Alleviating heat stress; Chapter 19 of Moran (2005) and Chapter 12 of Moran (2012a)
- Housing systems; Chapter 13 of Moran (2012a) and Chapter 7 of Moran (2012b)
- Key Performance Indicators of SHD herd performance; Chapter 14 of Moran (2009a)
- Communicating with the calf; Chapter 12 of Moran (2012b).

For the sake of brevity, when referring to farm operators and managers, this book uses the male possessive noun and pronoun, this does not necessarily assume them only to be men. In many situations, the description could apply equally to the farming women who make key management decisions.

It is not easy to write a book about small holder tropical dairy farming in which every fact is relevant to every reader. What is of most importance to the actual farmer may not be the most crucial fact for the educator of technical or university level students or the dairy adviser who chooses to read this book. Furthermore, tropical dairy farms take many forms ranging from very small holdings with fewer than five milking cows who are all hand milked, to larger operations with say 50 milking cows that are milked using 'bucket milkers'; these could be all owned by the one farmer or constitute a colony farm with many farmers owning small herds. Although grazing the milking herd is a rare feature of most tropical farms, the larger ones, with adequate land may be able to graze their dry cows or yearling heifers. Herd dynamics in a grazing situation can be very different to those in the confines of a shed, particularly one based on tie stalls. In future years, farmers may expand and be able to incorporate a milking parlour with fixed in line milking equipment. In fact virtually all sustainable dairy farms grow in the medium to long term, so for today's farmer with 10 cows or fewer who may become tomorrow's farmer with 30 or 50 cows, his knowledge of and practices to optimise cow behaviour with its consequential impact on their wellbeing, will need to be updated. This book, although not aiming to be 'all things to all people' has been written for a very diverse audience, so there will be technical aspects that are less relevant for some readers.

It is quite likely that many SHD (and even large-scale) farmers would find this book too technical and difficult to comprehend. In the first place, if English is not their mother tongue and unless they were well educated and/or travelled, very few would fully understand the English language. In the second place, the book is not simply a practical guide of how to ensure good stock welfare. Rather, it is a technical manual about:

- How modern day dairy cows evolved from their wild ancestors.
- What are natural behaviour patterns of cattle, how did they evolve in response to the changing management of dairy stock and how can we recognise abnormal behaviour?
- Since animals use different mechanisms to communicate, how do humans understand their needs? How do we interpret the many signals that they give out every day and what do we need to do to maintain their wellbeing under the constraints of commercial livestock farming?
- What is cow comfort and how do we measure it?
- How should we address animal welfare in current dairy production systems and how should this differ between countries and societies that farm dairy cattle for their milk and meat?
- How can good animal welfare best become profitably integrated into SHD systems in tropical Asia?

In other words, the book provides the theory as well as the practice behind the observations arising from poor stock welfare practices so farmers and advisers can understand the reasons why these practices need to be improved, that is 'why unacceptable things happen' and 'how they should be changed' to ensure they do not happen again.

1.3   Small holder dairy development in tropical Asia

SHD farmers supply over 80% of the annual global 240 billion litres of milk, with average herd sizes often as small as one to five milking cows. The Asia–Pacific region has seen the world's highest growth in demand for milk and dairy products. Total consumption has doubled over the last 30 years, contributing to more than 60% of the total increases in global consumption. For example in SE Asia, per capita milk consumption is expected to rise from the current 10 to 12 kg/hd/yr to 19 to 20 kg/hd/yr by the year 2020 (Delgardo *et al.* 2003). This 3% per annum growth will lead to a total milk consumption of 12 million tonnes/yr by 2020, which Delgardo *et al.* (2003) predicts will require 9 million tonnes milk/yr net imports to satisfy; this is up from 4.7 million tonnes milk/yr imported in 2000. Therefore by 2020, SE Asia will only be producing 25% of its milk requirements.

Such growing demands, prompted by higher incomes and increasing urbanisation, have combined with economic reforms and market liberalisation policies to heighten the import dependency of many countries in the region, where such imports have nearly doubled over the past decade. Asia has become increasingly dependent on highly competitive, but ever increasingly volatile, global dairy commodity markets. With production falling short of consumption gains, there has been a threefold increase in the importation of milk and dairy products.

Table 1.1 presents FAOSTAT (2010) data from 19 countries in South and East Asia on the numbers of dairy cows and milking buffalo and their total annual milk production, together with their changes in self-sufficiency over the last 10 years or so. To give an idea of the role of dairy products in their diet, the per capita consumption of all dairy products is also included in this table. These range from extremes of Pakistan (over 170 kg/capita/yr) to Laos (with only 2 kg/capita/yr).

For more detailed information on changes in the size and production of national dairy herds, the reader is referred to Chapter 3 in Moran (2009a). With regard to changes in self-sufficiency of milk and dairy products, several countries have maintained close to 100% self-sufficiency, while others have been unable to maintain previous levels of self-sufficiency because demand has greatly exceeded supply. Others have minimum levels that have hardly changed over the last 10 years.

The relevance of these data to this book is that most Asian countries that rely heavily on imported dairy products have active government policies to increase domestic milk production, often through importing large numbers of breeding stock. These animals are usually exotic heifers, either unbred or up to 5 months pregnant, in that they originate from temperate dairy industries where they have been reared on pasture in a largely climatically comfortable environment. Upon arrival, they then have to adapt to all the constraints of tropical SHD farming, such as high temperatures and humidities, limited quantities of poor to moderate quality feed and the vastly different rearing environment of a low investment system with limited to no grazing and a small cowshed. Changes in animal behaviour clearly indicate that this adaptation period can be quite traumatic and

Table 1.1. The size and self-sufficiency of selected Asian dairy industries in 2010.

	Total dairy consumption (kg/capita/yr) [2009 data]	Dairy cow population (000 head)	Buffalo population (000 head)	Total annual milk production (Kt or million kg/yr)	Self-sufficiency in milk (%)		
					2000	2005	2009
South Asia							
Afghanistan	–	3500	–	1401	100	100	100
Bangladesh	20.2	4059	90	866	74.7	66.7	70.5
India	72.2	44 900	37 131	117 253	100	100	100
Nepal	43.0	974	1291	1495	99.1	98.6	98.0
Pakistan	171.9	10 493	11 864	34 716	99.5	99.8	99.8
Sri Lanka	35.9	251	90	209	32.9	24.7	33.8
East Asia							
China	30.0	12 298	5706	39 136	87.0	91.8	95.1
N Korea	4.5	36	–	95	100	91.2	84.4
Japan	76.5	1000	–	7720	79.8	80.4	81.2
Mongolia	150.5	623	–	243	99.2	96.4	96.7
S Korea	22.9	186	–	2073	90.7	86.1	82.2
SE Asia							
Cambodia	4.3	137	–	27	48.5	52.1	33.4
Indonesia	11.5	597	–	840	37.6	31.9	30.0
Laos	2.2	35	–	7	26.5	22.5	35.2
Malaysia	36.7	147	10	74	3.3	3.5	6.1
Myanmar	29.0	2600	540	1387	83.0	85.6	92.2
Philippines	13.3	6	–	10	0.7	0.8	1.1
Thailand	21.9	285	–	851	28.8	45.5	50.3
Vietnam	11.5	133	32	341	19.5	19.6	30.6

lengthy, up to 6 months according to experienced small holder farmers. This is exacerbated by the often different standards of acceptable practices of stock welfare on their new home farm (see Figure 1.3).

There is a group of Asian countries with low per capita milk consumption and low self-sufficiencies and these are likely to be the ones with most proactive dairy heifer importation programs. These include Philippines, Indonesia, Thailand, Malaysia, Vietnam, Cambodia and Laos.

1.4 What do dairy cows really want?

While many of the welfare issues discussed in this book relate to the herd, it is important to remember that the welfare of an individual animal is important. With that in mind, Bos *et al.* (2009) list nine key factors in any dairy husbandry system that help reduce any negative impacts on dairy cow welfare:

- Resting space: provide at least one spacious resting spot for each cow so they can all rest at once if they want.

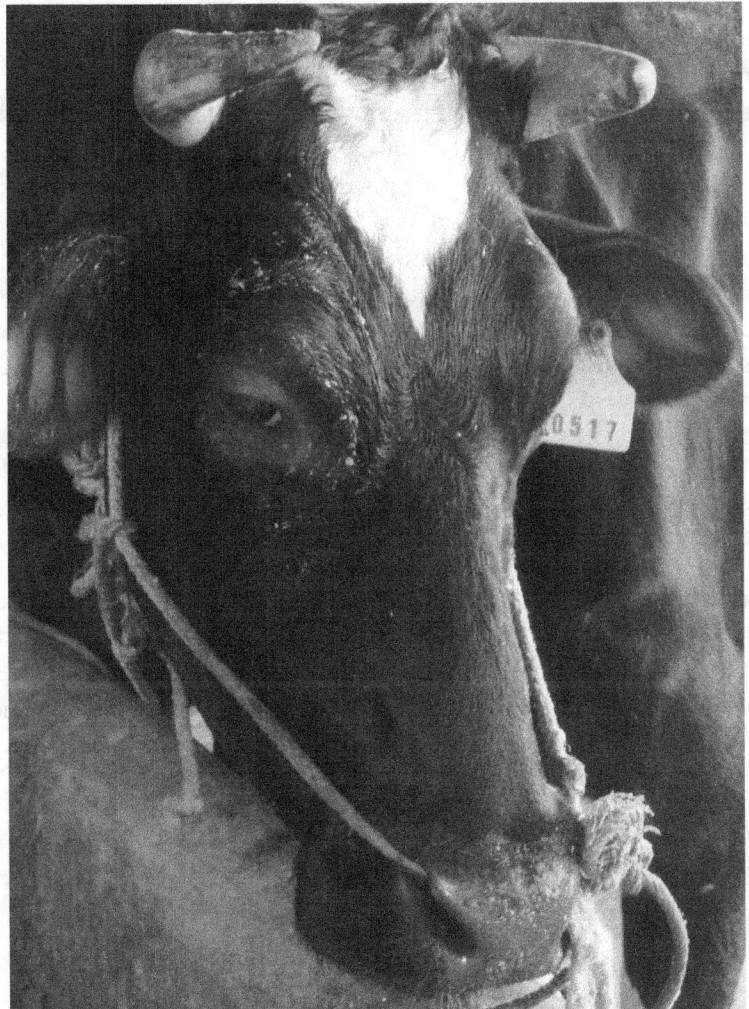

Figure 1.3: The typical method of nasal tethering a milking cow on small holder Asian dairy farms.

- Feed and water: you must provide feed that will enable the cow to maintain her body functions and produce milk. A continuous supply of fresh water is also a crucial requirement.
- Space to perform natural behaviours: cows need to be able to perform natural, healthy behaviours and freely move within the area and within the herd.
- Calm and predictable handling by people will reduce fear and improve milk production.
- No negative stimuli such as leakage of current and cow trainers (electric wires placed on top of free stalls): negative stimuli will cause (chronic) stress which adversely influences health and welfare.

- An environment without obstacles is needed for cows while getting up, lying down and during resting. Cows also require the opportunity to be able to lie down at some distance from other cows: they like to lie down in the way they would in the pasture. They want their own personal space, but may still like to lie close together.
- A comfortable climate: this is one with a Temperature Humidity Index below 71, which is equivalent to 27°C at 30% relative humidity or 24°C at 70% humidity (Moran 2005 and Appendix 1), and so avoiding heat stress.
- Passage ways and feeding areas with a non-slip, dry and clean floor without sudden changes in the level, slope or texture: if the floor is too smooth, cows may slip, if too rough, they may damage their hooves. Uneven, wet or dirty floors are detrimental to leg and hoof health.
- Sufficient light during the day and dark conditions for rest at night: cows must be able to see their surroundings properly, so they can recognise their herd mates, explore their surroundings or interact with their companions. Lighting in the day of more than 200 lux is recommended.

Providing all these prerequisites will ensure a happy, contented and productive herd. As will be outlined in the coming chapters, animal welfare is closely tied to the health and productivity of cows too, making it important to the producer from several different angles. The importance of these requirements and how they contribute to good welfare and production will be explained in the subsequent chapters.

2

Cow welfare

This chapter presents an introduction to animal welfare, specifically for dairy cattle.

The main points of this chapter

- An animal is in a good state (that is, its welfare is good) if it is healthy, comfortable, well nourished, safe, able to express innate behaviour, and if it is not suffering from negative states such as pain, fear and distress.
- Good animal welfare requires disease prevention and veterinary treatment, appropriate shelter, management, nutrition, humane handling, transport and eventually, humane slaughter.
- Examples of issues creating poor welfare on farms include morbidity and mortality, the existence of abnormal behaviours, poor housing, lameness, heat stress, tethering, painful husbandry procedures and poor calf management.

The welfare of an animal relates primarily to its ability to cope, both with its external environment – such as housing, handling by humans, weather and the presence of other animals, and with its internal environment – such as specific injuries or illnesses and nutritional status. Welfare refers not only to the internal and external environments of animals, but how they feel. These feelings can be negative, including pain, fear and hunger, or they can be positive, including calmness and happiness.

The health and welfare of an animal are closely linked with the health status of an animal influencing its welfare, and its welfare influencing its health. Cattle kept in poor or chronically stressful conditions are more susceptible to disease, which usually reduces the quality of their end products. As well as a reduction in production, cattle in poor welfare states can be more susceptible to zoonotic diseases, such as tuberculosis, which can be transmitted in milk to humans. Cattle with illnesses and injuries, particularly chronic ones, are classified as having poor welfare. Production can also be included in this relationship, with healthy and contented cattle being more productive.

This three-way interaction is a complex one, for example the European Food Safety Authority (2009) states that long-term genetic selection for high milk yield is a major factor contributing to poor welfare. In particular, this refers to health problems in dairy cows such as lameness, mastitis, metabolic instability and longevity. In other words, we breed cows to produce more and more milk at the expense of their welfare. This is particularly relevant to poorly resourced dairy farmers and/or those who do not fully understand the impact these genetically selected high milk yields can have on the energy demands of cows. These nutritional deficits then infringe on their welfare, making them more susceptible to metabolic and reproductive problems.

While the welfare of an animal is a dynamic thing, dependent on changes in the animal's health and environment, some simple, fundamental features will guarantee good welfare. These are: good hygiene, having continuous access to clean water, stable social groups and the provision of preventative veterinary care. This chapter details what animal welfare is, the factors that affect it and how we can improve it.

2.1 What is animal welfare?

Animal welfare refers to an animal's physical and mental state, and how it is coping with its situation. According to the World Organization for Animal Health (Office International des Epizooties 2013) an animal is in a good state of welfare if it is healthy, comfortable, well nourished, safe, able to express its innate behaviour, and is not suffering from negative states such as pain, fear and distress. Good animal welfare requires disease prevention and veterinary treatment, appropriate shelter, management, nutrition, humane handling, transport and eventually, humane slaughter. This definition and issues that surround it are the basis of this book. As well as cattle, these concepts about animal welfare apply to all animals that interact with humans, including agricultural, companion, circus and zoo animals and those used in science.

While this definition is accepted internationally, what people interpret to be acceptable animal welfare can be influenced by many factors including personal values, religion, nationality, gender, previous experiences, age, socio-economic status, education and so on. Throughout both this chapter and this book we describe dairy cattle welfare to levels that are recognised internationally and are based on scientific research.

Animal welfare is directly related to the health of animals, sustainable livestock management and market assurances. As farm animal welfare is largely part of good animal and farm management, paying close attention to their day-to-day management is one of the most important factors when determining acceptable welfare.

Concern for and assessment of animal welfare generally falls into three categories (Fraser *et al.* 1997):

- Is the animal functioning well?
- Is the animal feeling well?
- Is the animal able to live a reasonably natural life?

The first category includes issues with the productivity and health of the animal, including whether or not it is free from illness and injury, and how well it is growing and producing. Concerns over whether an animal is feeling well refer to the animal's emotional state, as it is widely agreed that animals can experience fundamental emotions. Animals in a negative emotional state may be in pain, distressed or hungry. Positive states experienced by animals may include the pleasure associated with play, or contentment as all their needs are being satisfied. The third key concern is whether the animal is able to live a relatively natural life and can express natural behaviour, for example, the ability to lie comfortably or move freely. While these second two categories are less commonly thought of in production animals, they are important to consider because of the strong relationships between emotional state, the inability to express natural behaviours, stress and production (von Keyserlingk *et al.* 2009).

2.2 Why animal welfare is important

Not only is it important to understand what welfare is, but we also need to know *why* it is of importance. Animal welfare is fundamentally linked to animal health and production (Moberg 2001). Both clinical and subclinical disease states will compromise the welfare of animals. For example, lameness causes a cow to feel pain, and as a result, this will impact on her ability to feed, rest, move and cope with other illnesses and stressful situations that she experiences. Poor welfare can also have a negative impact on the health of a cow. Stressful situations, such as negative treatment by a stockperson or ongoing aggressive interactions with other animals in the herd, will result in physiological and behavioural changes in the animal that are aimed at helping it to deal with the stress. If the stressor is prolonged, becoming chronic, these physiological responses can impact upon the immunity of the cow, making her more susceptible to disease. Poor welfare is also linked to reduced productivity, inhibiting the capacity for the cow to reproduce, reducing milk yields and body condition. For example, illness can reduce feed intake and divert resources from production to fighting infection. Cattle that experience fear during handling will also have reduced milk yields. More details on the significance of this interaction and related behaviours are detailed in Chapter 4.

As well as the direct influence it has on animals and their health as part of sustainable livestock production systems, public perceptions of farm animal welfare issues have the potential to markedly affect the security/sustainability of livestock industries. Nationally and internationally, these societal pressures are playing increasingly significant roles in determining how animals are managed and products are marketed, while scientific findings assist development of welfare assessment, practice and improvement.

2.3 Common welfare issues on dairy farms

Generally, animal welfare is considered to be 'good' if the animals are healthy, comfortable, well nourished and safe and are not suffering from unpleasant states such as pain, fear and distress. Cows also need to be able to express basic behaviours including lying, turning around, scratching and displaying social behaviours to a reasonable degree. This idea of good welfare includes aspects from all three categories listed in Section 2.1. In contrast to these positive states are the environments or situations where cows are not functioning well, feeling well or able to have a reasonably natural life.

2.3.1 Morbidity and mortality

On farms, morbidity (sickness) and mortality (death) are the most fundamental welfare issues. High levels of illness and any subsequent deaths relate to the poor functioning of animals, and can also include the other two broad welfare categories, particularly if the illness is chronic and the animal has suffered for an extended period of time, or the illness is acute and painful.

2.3.2 Behavioural abnormalities

When a cow is in a state of poor welfare, her behaviour will indicate this. These behavioural changes may include a modified gait, signalling hoof pain and lameness and the duration of lying bouts and the position the cow takes to indicate the comfort of her environment. Social behaviours, or a lack thereof, can indicate issues with the ability to express normal behaviours. The existence of stereotypic behaviours, defined as a repeated sequence of behaviours that has no apparent purpose, is the result of frustrations and the inability to perform normal behaviours. Full details on normal and abnormal behaviours are presented in Chapter 4.

2.3.3 Housing

Housing can have a significant influence on the welfare of cows, affecting all three welfare categories. Whether housed in tie stalls, free stalls or open lounging systems, in order to maximise performance and ensure satisfactory standards of welfare, the accommodation must provide for the animal's basic needs. As an absolute minimum, the housing must provide a comfortable, clean, and well-drained dry lying area that provides shelter from adverse weather. The space provided should be enough that the animal can express behaviours that will allow it to be comfortable including standing, turning, scratching and lying. Housing systems should also allow the animal to move without risk of injury. The provision of an environment that fulfils these criteria is a common theme in quantitative measures of dairy cow welfare, highlighting its importance.

Poor housing not only affects the day-to-day comfort of the cow, but also has flow-on effects to their health. Cows at pasture, which is one of the most comfortable environments for them, choose to lie down for 12 to 14 h each day. Reduced lying time is an indication of an uncomfortable lying area or potentially another compromised welfare situation, for example, increased vigilance and fear, with cattle feeling unsafe in their home environment. If cows spend less time lying down, they are likely to spend more time standing in loafing or feeding areas, which can adversely affect hoof health, leading to conditions like lameness (see Figure 2.1). Furthermore, housing and management influence the likelihood of animals experiencing heat stress, which is a significant issue in the tropics (see Figures 2.2 and 2.3).

The provision of pasture has been linked with reduced levels of mastitis, reduced levels of lameness and faster recovery from these issues (von Keyserlingk et al. 2009). When animals are allowed to spend time in an environment they prefer, their affective state is assumed to be more positive because they are provided with a situation they desire. Cows have a preference for lying at pasture rather than indoors, indicating they find it more comfortable. While cows prefer to be indoors, rather than in full sun when it is hot, providing cows with access to both environments will ensure positive welfare. Cows with access to pasture also display abnormal behaviours less frequently and more normal social behaviours than do cows continually kept indoors. Providing cows with pasture access then helps to promote good welfare across the three welfare categories and improves the productivity of the animal by reducing disease and aiding recovery.

Chapter 7, 'Cow comfort', is dedicated to types of housing systems, the benefits and disadvantages of each for a cow's health and welfare, and ways to assess the appropriateness of this housing.

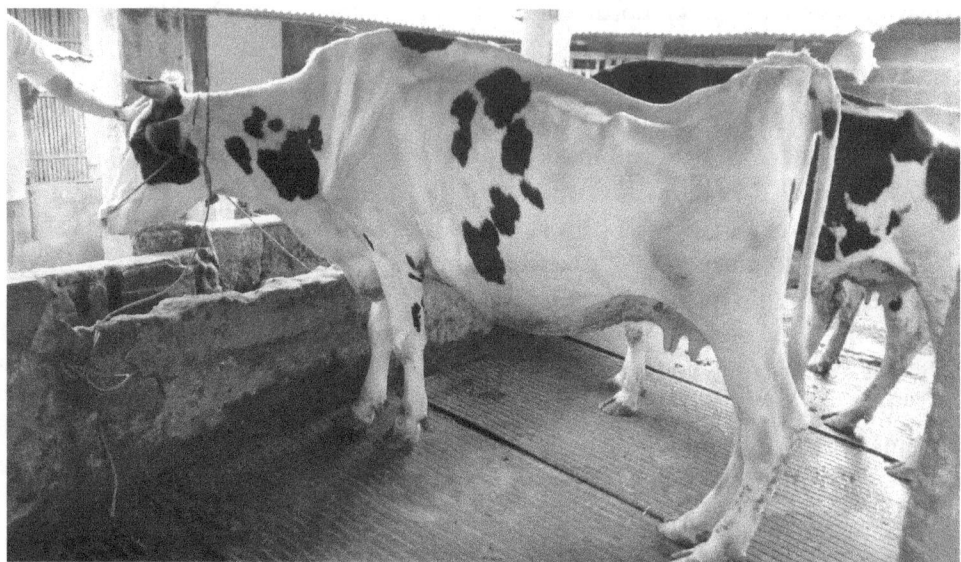

Figure 2.1: An old cow with permanent skeleton deformities as a result of a lifetime of tethering.

2.3.4 Lameness

Lameness is a major problem on dairy farms, both from the point of animal welfare and farm profits. Lameness can result from infectious diseases or from lesions/injury to the hoof. Management factors have a significant influence on the number and severity of lameness cases. The design of facilities, including uneven concrete floors and uncomfortable stalls with no bedding, are important risk factors for lameness, as is the structural integrity of the cow's hoof. Stockperson ability to identify lameness is also very influential, with farmers/stockpeople only recognising 40 to 50% of lameness problems, and only being able to identify these issues when they become severe (von Keyserlingk *et al.* 2009). These cases of lameness are often well advanced once they are identified for the first time, meaning that the animal is suffering for a long period of time and making the condition difficult to treat. Lameness can be even more difficult to detect in tethered systems and often remains as a shifting lameness condition, misinterpreted or undetected and untreated. Factors that increase the likelihood of a cow developing lameness are discussed in Chapter 5. Methods of identifying and scoring this common issue are presented in Chapter 6.

2.3.5 Heat stress

Heat stress can be common, particularly in high yielding cows in the tropics. Cows experiencing heat stress will show a variety of symptoms including discomfort and distress, that affect their wellbeing. An increased core body temperature, increased

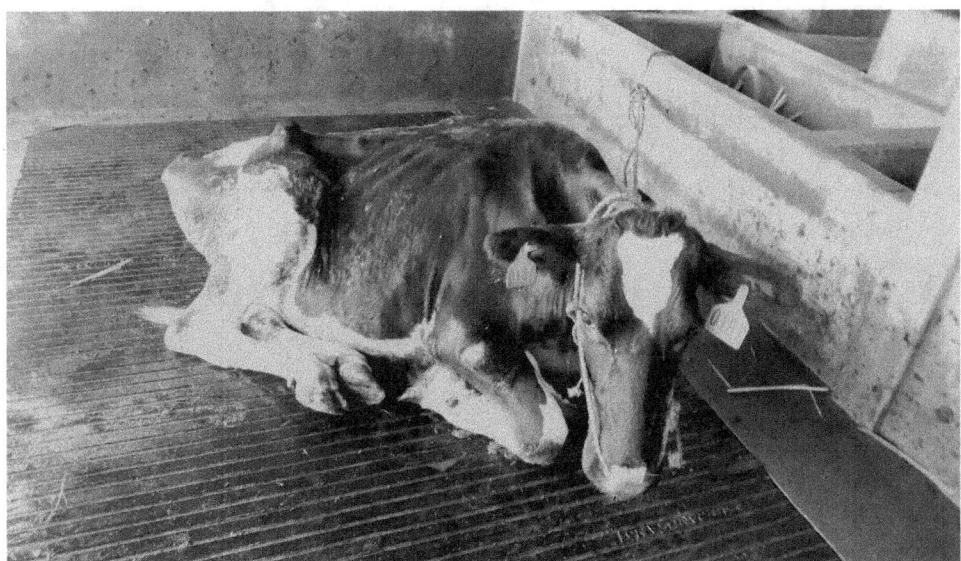

Figure 2.2: A milking cow in very poor health, probably suffering from poor management and welfare as well as disease.

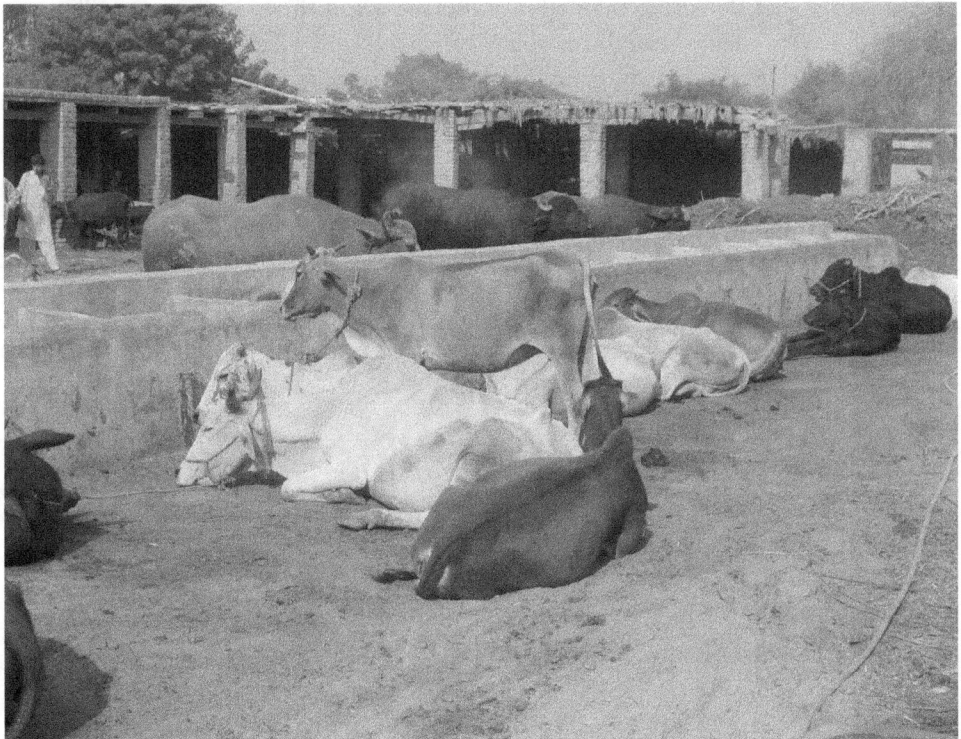

Figure 2.3: Tethering stock under the tropical sun is poor stock welfare.

respiration rate, drooling and sweating are all signs of their functioning being compromised. General abnormal behaviours include reduced feed intake, agitated and restless behaviour, and standing for long periods of time, rather than lying down. Weather and climate are the driving factors behind heat stress. However, with the correct management and facility design, heat stress can be dealt with effectively, reducing the physiological stress on the animal. Details on the detection and management of heat stress can be found in Chapters 5 and 6.

2.3.6   Tethering

Tethering is a common practice in Asian dairy farms. This type of environment can cause significant welfare issues as it is closely associated with high levels of disease, discomfort and abnormal behaviours in dairy cows (Blaszak 2011). Animals that are continuously tethered are more likely to be dirty than animals that are kept in tie free housing (Figures 2.4 and 2.5). This is important as dirty cows have a much greater risk of mastitis and lameness, and are more likely to pass diseases on to calves as well as zoonotic diseases to humans through their milk. Cows in tie stalls also display both restless behaviours and abnormal behaviours more frequently than cows that are not tethered (Figure 2.6). Several sections in this book have been dedicated to these important topics. Further details on health and welfare issues that are generated by tethering are outlined in Chapter 7. The issue of abnormal behaviour and examples of this are provided in Chapter 4. Details on why clean and comfortable housing are important are outlined in Chapter 5 and ways to identify the cleanliness of cows are outlined in Chapter 6.

The welfare of tethered cows can be greatly improved by maintaining a clean environment, ensuring that the flooring they have is comfortable, providing water *ad libitum*, and giving them access to pasture and/or the ability to walk around freely for a few hours each day. These simple changes can significantly improve the milk yields, health and welfare of animals. For example, in a study with shedded cows in Pakistan, the provision of water *ad libitum* compared to only twice daily, increased milk yields by up to 1.5 L/cow/day.

2.3.7   Painful husbandry practices

Some management practices cause pain to animals. These practices should be avoided where possible, or if they are necessary, they should be performed by a well-trained technician or veterinarian. It is important to consider ways to limit the pain an animal may experience during these processes. Pain can be significantly alleviated by the provision of pain relief. When pain relief cannot be administered, some methods are considered to be less painful than others. Recommendations on both situations are outlined below.

Tail docking can be a common practice performed on dairy farms that causes significant pain to the animal, but there is no evidence of practical benefit. In the short term, the procedure of tail docking causes significant pain to the cow along with leaving an open wound. In the long term, this can lead to chronic pain, the same way a person with an amputation experiences pain (known as phantom limb pain). Tail docking is practised because it is thought to improve hygiene of the udder, but there is no research to support this (Schreiner and Ruegg 2002). Tail docking, therefore, is an example of a practice that causes unnecessary pain to the animal, without any management benefit and so it should not be performed.

Dehorning and disbudding are common painful husbandry practices performed on dairy farms. Horns on a cow can pose a threat to the farmer and other cows that the horned animal interacts with, therefore dehorning is a necessary management practice. The age at which horn removal is conducted and the method used have an effect on the amount of pain and distress the animal experiences (Stafford and Mellor 2005a). There are several methods by which horns can be removed. Disbudding is carried out on young calves, before the horn has actually started to grow. Dehorning is the removal of the horn and horn-producing tissue. Cautery disbudding uses a hot iron to remove and burn the horn bud. This technique is suitable for calves 12 weeks or younger, and causes the least pain to the animal and the smallest wound area. This is the recommended method and timing of horn removal. While cautery disbudding is the best practice method for disbudding, it can be difficult to perform in SHD situations.

Caustic disbudding uses a paste to remove the horn bud. Along with being painful, this type of disbudding can cause irritation to the surrounding areas of the skin, can damage the eye if the paste runs down the calf's face, and can also cause irritation to other animals that the calf comes into contact with. As a result, calves should be housed by themselves in the hours after the paste has been applied, and the dehorned area must be kept dry. Pain management for caustic disbudding is difficult to manage and so is not recommended.

Amputation dehorning, conducted on animals at a later age, creates a wound that can open the frontal sinus of the animal. This procedure causes extensive pain, long wound healing times and significantly reduced weight gains. It also creates a large risk of infection. Pain relief using both a local anaesthetic and non-steroidal anti-inflammatory are highly recommended in this particular situation, and all animals treated with these alleviation methods have shown indicators of a reduced pain response. The wound site will also bleed significantly and clamps or tourniquets should be used to reduce bleeding.

Castration is less common in dairying than it is in beef production, as bull calves are usually sold or slaughtered before they reach sexual maturity. In small holder systems, it is more common to keep bull calves until they reach heavier slaughter weights, and so castration can be a usual procedure. There are several different methods for castration, and the age of the calf has a significant influence on which method is most effective and least painful (Stafford and Mellor 2005b).

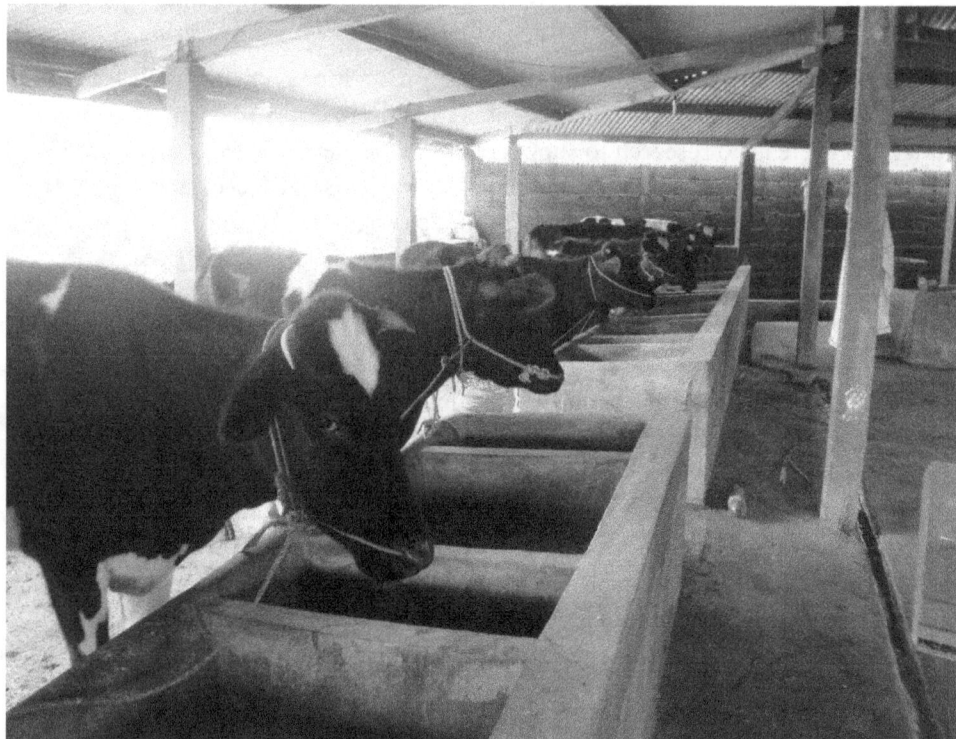

Figure 2.4: Permanent tethering: typical management of too many cows on tropical small holder farms.

Calves at a younger age display less pain during castration than older animals. For calves younger than 3 months of age, rubber ring castration has a high success rate and has the best welfare outcome for the animal. As it does not involve a surgical procedure, there is no blood loss or evidence of acute pain, compared to calves castrated with a knife. Calves 3 months or younger are much easier to handle than older animals, making the castration procedure safer for both the handlers and the animal. Rubber ring castration is ineffective on older cattle. For these animals, surgical castration is the best option. It is recommended that older cattle be castrated using an emasculator, as this cuts the blood supply as well as severing the testes, and so reduces blood loss. It is strongly recommended that surgical castration be performed on older cattle following the administration of both a local anaesthetic and a non-steroidal anti-inflammatory (ketoprofen), in order to minimise pain.

2.3.8 Calf management

The provision of the right environment, food and health care to a calf are vitally important to their subsequent productivity and lifespan as an adult. From birth, colostrum needs to be fed and followed by mastitis-free milk in appropriate volumes to ensure the good health and growth of calves. Other factors that need to be managed appropriately to ensure good welfare and growth include care and

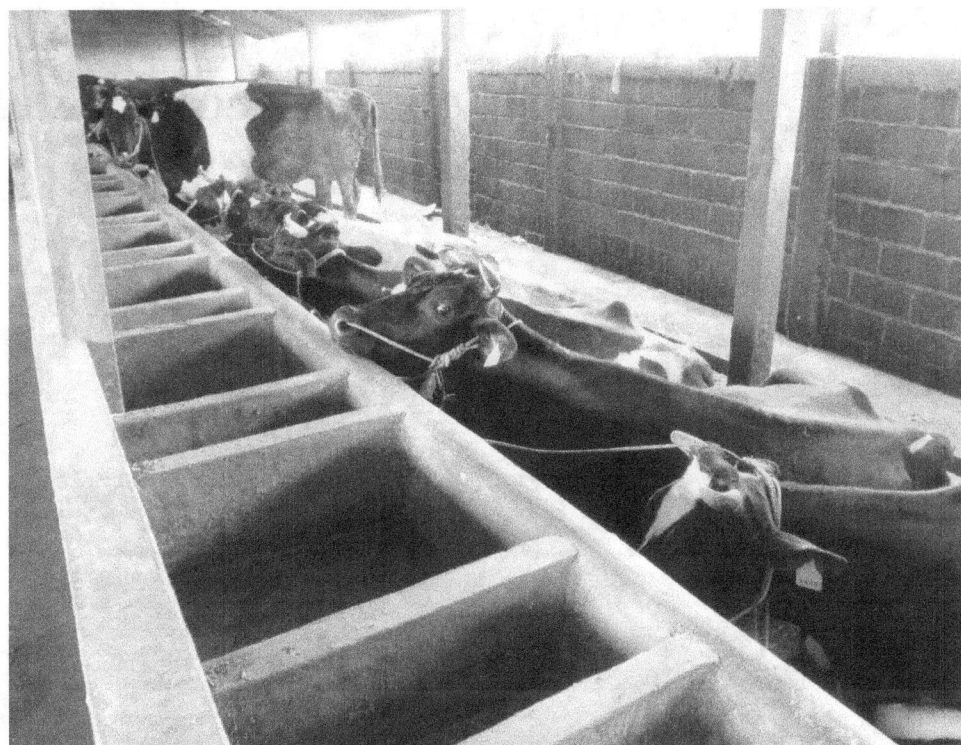

Figure 2.5: Permanent tethering restricts the animal's ability to rest comfortably.

monitoring of the newborn calf, the appropriate provision of forage for rumen development and a graduated approach to weaning. A detailed manual on the effective rearing of calves on tropical SHD farms is freely available (Moran 2012b).

Along with appropriate feeding and management to ensure good health, the environment in which calves are kept significantly affects their welfare and development. It is recommended that calves be housed in a way that they can easily stand, lie, turn around, rest comfortably and have visual contact with other calves (Vasseur *et al.* 2012). Further to this, housing calves in pairs or small groups has been associated with play in calves, which is an indicator of positive welfare and allows them to develop normal social behaviours. Importantly, keeping calves in small groups has not been linked to increased incidences of disease, which is a common argument against group housing (Svensson *et al.* 2003).

2.4 Animal welfare resources and international regulatory agencies

An example list of government and non-government agencies within Australia that are involved in cattle welfare, together with their websites, are included as Appendix 6. A total of 178 countries are currently members of the World

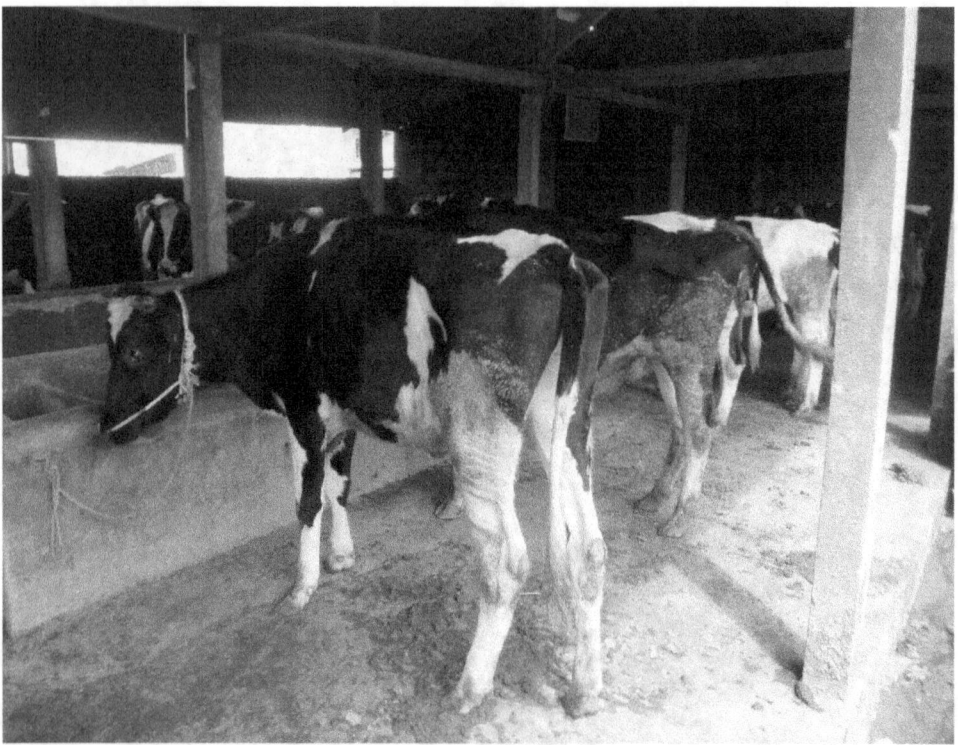

Figure 2.6: Permanently tethered dairy heifers are forced to lie down on hard concrete.

Association for Animal Health or the Office International des Epizooties (OIE) and the OIE website is included in Appendix 6. The OIE are in the process of producing animal welfare standards for animals used by humans. The OIE currently have guidelines that cover transport and slaughter that can directly apply to dairy cattle welfare. These standards act as a guideline from which management strategies and policies can be developed. At the time of printing of this book, work on a code for dairy cattle welfare had commenced.

3

The implications of cattle domestication

This chapter presents an insight into domestication, such as the timelines and impact on natural cattle behaviour.

The main points of this chapter

- When domestication began, the human–animal relationship developed towards a symbiosis in which humans provided food and protection from predators in exchange for animal products (food and fur) and power.
- By keeping and selecting cattle for commercial production, we have reduced their longevity.
- Humans have modified the genotype of cattle for their own benefit more than any other species of domestic livestock and, in the process of this modification, we have often improved their welfare.
- Our modification of the cattle genotype has enabled us to keep them in a wide variety of conditions and environments. Even in environments where many people would consider that cattle are not well adapted, they still produce economic quantities of milk or grow at commercially acceptable rates.
- It is believed that selection of behavioural characteristics played a very important part in the early stages of cattle domestication.

- The greatest impact of housing on the behaviour and welfare of cattle is on their social structure, since it is necessary to bring them into much closer contact than would have been the case if they were living outdoors.
- Another major effect of housing is on their predisposition to specific diseases, such as lameness.
- Cattle have had to change their behaviour patterns to adapt to social and human influences.

3.1 How modern day cattle evolved

Throughout the history of the human species, animals have played an important part in human life, and vice versa. In the early hunter-gatherer/nomadic cultures, animals were viewed as prey, but also as dangerous predators. The same holds true for the animals' perspective as some species considered humans as predators, some as prey. When domestication began, the human–animal relationship developed towards a symbiosis in which humans provided food and protection from predators in exchange for animal products (food and fur) and power. Domestication can be defined as an evolutionary process by which a population of captive animals adapt to man and the environment he provides; this occurs over many generations through a combination of genetic changes and environmental experiences recurring each generation (Price 1998). Domestication is more than just taming, as it also includes goal-orientated breeding programs in captivity. In essence, it is a system in which the breeding, care and feeding of animals is completely under the control of humans. Like their human counterparts, domesticated animals now take on a wide variety of roles, with cattle the most diverse of all production animals, being suppliers of draught power, food and also animals connected with temples.

Fossilised cattle remains have been found in India dating back 2 million years, while in France, cattle drawings in caves have been found dating from 15 000 years ago. Based on archaeological remains, cattle were first domesticated in south-west Turkey ~8000 years ago with the more drought tolerant, humped (Zebu) cattle developed in Iran some 7000 years ago. However, more recent blood analyses have dated the origins of cattle to 500 000 years, long before modern humans were involved (Albright and Arave 1997). Cattle have been used in human cultures primarily as draught animals, as sources of ceremonial objects, meat, milk, leather, fertiliser, by-products and as trusting companions and possessions. Cattle were first selected for worship, because of their crescent-shaped horns that represented different phases of the moon. Their next key role was as draught animals to pull carts in temple ceremonies and in sacrificial rites, hence their selection for a quiet disposition and the appropriate horn shape. Much later, their role as suppliers of food and other by-products became the main concerns. Almost all great civilisations were built by people with a bull-cow culture, compared to those with only sheep and goats. Not only were they a greater source of meat and milk than pigs, sheep and goats which had been domesticated earlier than cattle, they were also the first draught animals to work the land during agricultural (grain growing) evolution. Some cattle became specialised dairy or specialised beef breeds while others were dual-purpose breeds supplying both these products. Physical work has always been a product but now horses and tractors have taken over this role. In many developing countries, cattle are still a sign of wealth and prestige.

Only in India has a major cow culture survived where cattle are still revered. All but two Indian states currently have laws strictly forbidding mistreatment or slaughter of cattle. Special cow nursing homes have even been established to take care of barren cows and those no longer able to work. Even in Singapore, the senior author has visited a dairy farm that daily supplies the local Hindu temple with fresh milk from a herd of ~30 milking cows, but also has a second herd of over 60 aging, dry and non pregnant cows that are maintained until their natural deaths. In such cases, religion and culture are considered more important than farm profits.

3.2   Impacts of domestication

During the domestication process, humans have provided the basic requirements such as food, water, a suitable environment, veterinary care and companionship, but have taken away the freedoms that cattle would have in the wild, such as choice of mate, companion, and feed and – of most importance – their freedom of movement. Furthermore, by keeping and selecting for commercial production, we have reduced their longevity, which would otherwise be as high as 20 to 25 years, for various reasons such as:

- Draught animals are culled when they become 'too old' because of the high demands of their work.
- Meat animals become less efficient in converting stock feed to saleable products and older cattle have lower growth rates and produce increasingly more fat in their carcasses.
- Milk animals are culled because of metabolic strain after only three or four lactations, or 6 or 7 years old, due to the impact of the stress of many lactations and the poor conditions that they are often kept in.

Humans have modified the genotype of cattle for their own benefit more than any other species of domestic livestock. In the process of this modification, many aspects of their welfare have improved. The ease with which cattle can coexist with humans is in marked contrast to other species that have not been as extensively domesticated. Training an animal to voluntarily walk to the milking parlour twice daily then stand still for up to 10 min is a perfect example of this level of domestication. Other species farmed for their saleable products such as deer, ostriches, mink and even sheep are more difficult to handle as many individuals often show high levels of aggression towards each other and their keepers. There have been attempts, largely unsuccessful, to domesticate gazelles, antelopes and even hyenas.

Through centuries of intensive selective breeding for milk production by humans, dairy cows have evolved to become one of the most efficient biological machines in the world. For example, within the Friesian breed, dairy cows in early lactation can produce up to seven times more animal protein each day than rapidly growing bulls. Dairy cows, averaging 25 L of milk per day, each produce 700 g/day of milk protein in contrast to the 100 g/day of carcass protein retained in rapidly growing Friesian bulls (Moran and Wood 1986).

As well as changing the basic anatomy of cattle through selection for meat or milk production, their dehorning is another evolutionary step in their domestication. The breeding of poll (hornless) beef and dairy cattle is now routine, as is the removal of vestigial horn 'buds' in calves. Without horns, cattle have become more compatible at the feed trough, in yards and at pasture, with less injury to each other and to humans. Hornless heifers spend more time eating and ruminating than do horned heifers (Albright and Arave 1997). When kept singly, hornless heifers gain more weight than horned heifers or than when kept in groups.

Our modification of the cattle genotype has enabled us to keep them in a wide variety of conditions and environments. Even in environments where many people would consider that cattle are not well adapted, they still produce economic quantities of milk or grow at commercially acceptable rates. It is argued, however, that this does not mean that such systems are justified just because the stock do not overtly manifest their difficulties in coping with the system. Cattle 'suffer in silence' partly due to the impact of domestication and partly due to the evolutionary forces pre-domestication. They are prey animals that graze in open grasslands and do not wish to attract attention to themselves by active vocalisation or other displays if they are having trouble coping with the environment.

The International Dairy Federation (IDF) (2008) have identified four stages of domestication of dairy cattle for human benefit and how these have impacted on their welfare:

1. In their wild state the animals expressed natural productivity but their welfare was not maximised because of predation, disease, lack of feed and other adverse natural events.
2. As they became domesticated and more of their needs were fulfilled through commercial farming, their production increased and their welfare improved

since all their basic needs were met along with protection from disease and shelter; this would then have been their point of maximal welfare.

3. Beyond this point, further efforts have been made to increase production and this starts to impinge on their welfare.

4. Ultimately there arrives a point at which the increased drive for production will reach or even exceed their biological limits and their welfare becomes poor.

Therefore, an excessive drive for very high production can result in a sharp decline in animal welfare below those of their wild counterparts unless adequate resources are provided to meet the demands of this increased production. IDF argue that Stage 4 may have already been reached in some systems of dairy farming. Poorly managed tropical small holder dairy (SHD) farming with genetically selected high producing dairy cows could be one such example.

3.3 Impacts on behaviour

The behaviour of domestic cattle has been extensively studied and it is believed that selection of behavioural characteristics played a very important part in the early stages of domestication. However, there are many problem behaviours that can contribute to reduced productive efficiencies and these will be discussed in more detail in the following chapters. Many have been derived from the artificial environment that cattle are often kept in, since these abnormalities are absent in extensively kept cattle. They often evolve when animals are unable to behave naturally. They are particularly common in hot, humid regions where heat stress reduces their resistance to such environmental constraints. Opportunities to modify the environment are always limited, unless productivity is greatly reduced.

These problem behaviours discussed in Chapter 4 include:

- excessive licking and sucking behaviour in calves
- mounting behaviour in steers
- tongue rolling, prepuce sucking and stereotypes in steers
- excessive licking and grooming in cows
- physical evidence of metabolic problems in digesting high carbohydrate feedstuffs.

3.3.1 Housing

Intensive housing has one of the greatest impacts on the behaviour and welfare of cattle (Figure 3.1). This situation alters their social structure, as they are kept in much closer contact than when they are housed extensively. Another major effect of housing is on their predisposition to specific diseases (Figure 3.2), such as lameness. However, cattle can adapt to a variety of housing systems, in that they can tolerate being housed individually or in small or large groups (Figure 3.3). Space availability can be reduced to little more than that required for the animal to stand up or lie down. A major part of domestication is to facilitate adaptation to housing. Such changes in the environment can result in abnormal stereotypic behaviour (repeated sequences of a behaviour that has no apparent purpose or benefit) that develop rapidly in intensively housed cattle with inadequate space and diet. Other non-stereotyped behaviours, such as intersuckling and excessive licking and grooming, are also indicative of deficiencies in the environment. Sometimes the housing causes a restriction on movement that is not conducive to good welfare for the animal but is for the benefit of the herdsperson. For example, stalled cattle may have a 'cow trainer' (electrified wires) placed above them to ensure that they move backwards when they arch their back to urinate or defecate, so the excreta is conveniently placed in the alleyway rather than on the bedding.

Temperature stressors can occur either inside or outside the housing. Inadequate ventilation and radiant heat load from a low roof are the most likely

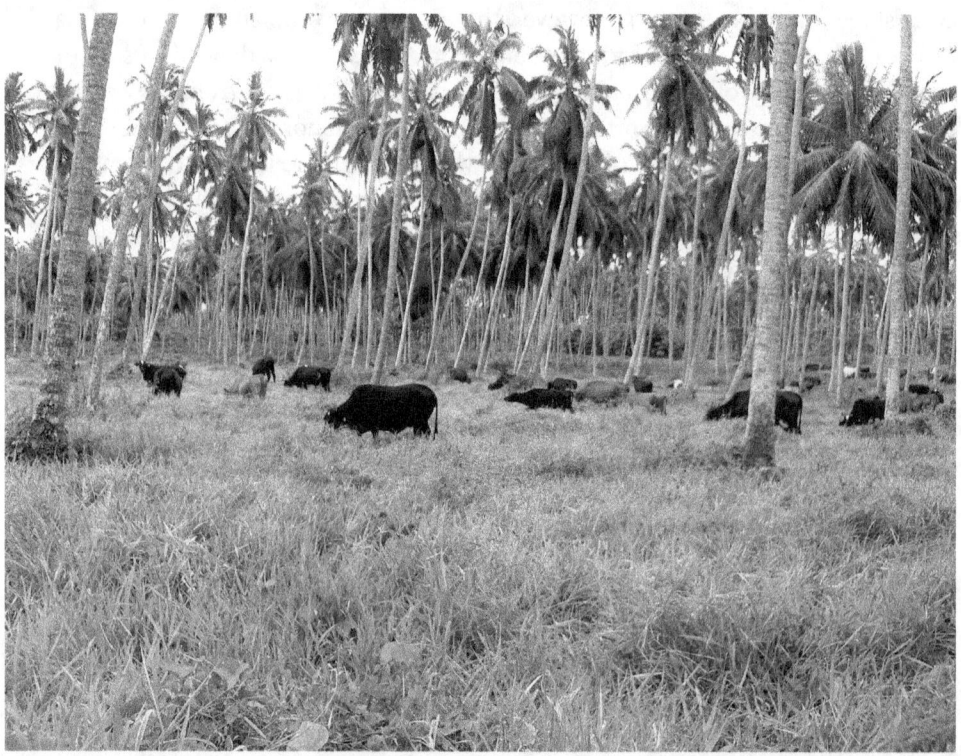

Figure 3.1: Rarely do milking cows have an opportunity to graze on tropical small holder farms.

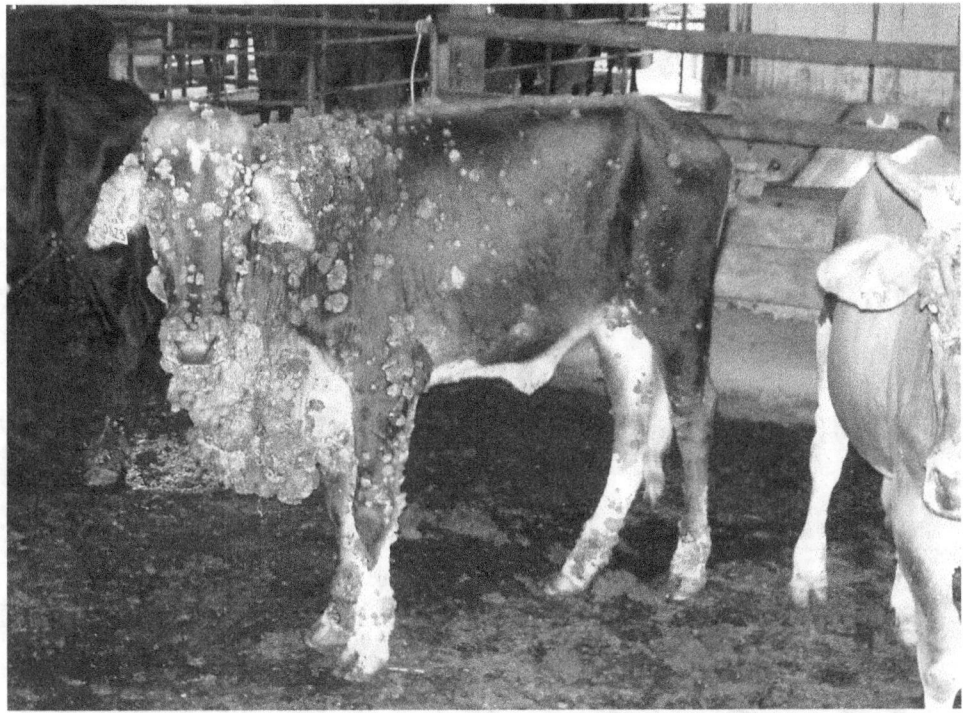

Figure 3.2: A dairy heifer suffering from severe skin infestation of papilloma virus. This is primarily the result of high density housing.

causes of heat stress. Outdoors, lack of shade is often a problem. Heat stress can be exacerbated because of the considerable heat of digestion occurring in the rumen. Cattle are also stressed by driving rain and will seek shelter, particularly avoiding facing the rain.

Stray electricity affects cattle more than humans. This stray voltage can originate from faulty equipment grounding, which often occurs in the corrosive environment of the cattle shed, or from a large voltage drop on the farm, which results in the supply being out of phase with the central power source.

3.3.2 Lameness

Much of the lameness in housed cattle is associated with cows walking or turning on hard or uneven concrete covered in slurry. The shock of regularly stepping on concrete, coupled with the softening of the hoof when the cow stands in slurry, can traumatise the hoof and lead to primary foot lesions.

Bad cubicle design may predispose cattle to lameness. Cows spend less time lying in small cubicles, cubicles with hard surfaces or cubicles with divisions that impede movement. Hock damage may occur as the animal lies down, especially on

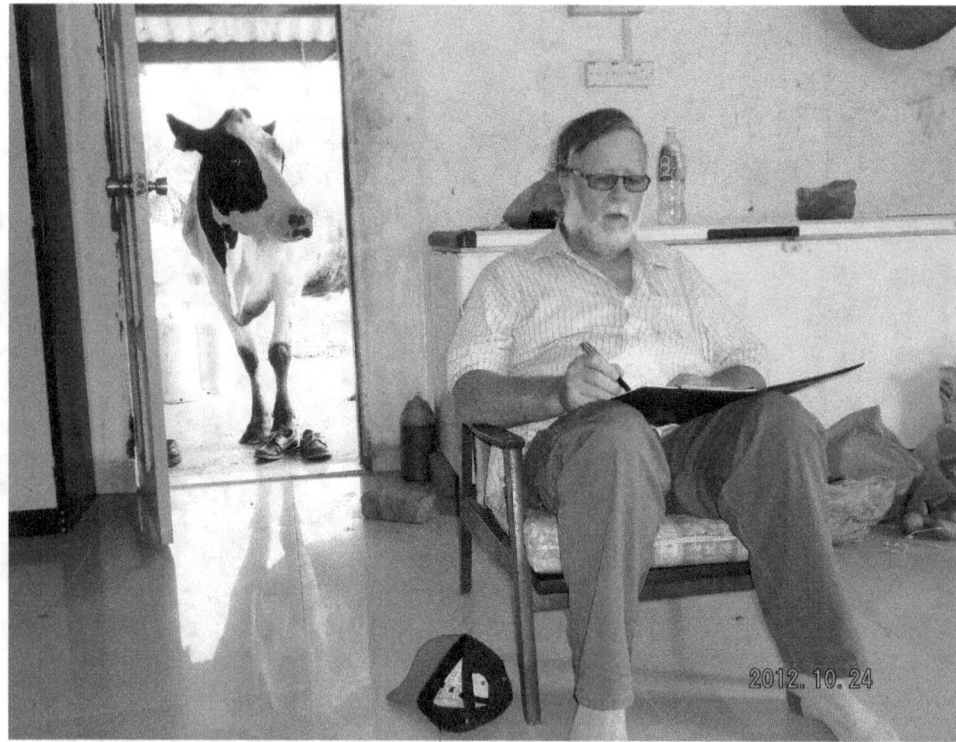

Figure 3.3: Milking cows can become very placid when well looked after.

abrasive surfaces. Stock lying on soft surfaces or in wide cubicles are less likely to experience this problem. However, if cubicles are too wide, cows may attempt to turn around and get stuck, particularly if they are inexperienced at lying in cubicles.

3.3.3 Social influences

The impact of social circumstances is much harder to define than that of other aspects of cow management. In the presence of a dominant cow, subordinate cows take evasive action. In a confined space, such as a shed, many escape attempts take place every day. Overt aggression is rare and an unsuccessful escape attempt is most likely to be met by a ritualised threat display. Social interaction between animals that is associated with aggression, including threatening and submissive behaviour, is referred to as agonistic behaviour. Unless food resources are limiting, there is little evidence that milk yield of subordinate cows is any less than of dominant cows. However, the movement of cows between different groups can reduce milk yield, and high stocking densities in dairy cow buildings can increase blood indicators of stress.

At pasture, dairy cows show evidence of increased vigilance when they are in groups of fewer than eight cows. Large groups in small paddocks or strip grazed cows will show more aggression than if they were grazed in a larger field. Competition for resources, such as food, may induce fighting between cows, but even then, damage to an individual is rare unless the cows are horned. Competition may be prevented by feeding concentrate at barriers in sheds with self-locking yokes.

Separation of cow and calf will stress some cows, particularly if the separation occurs after a substantial period together. Initially after separation the cow makes attempts to reunite with the calf, through increased locomotion and vocalisation and even breaking of separation fences. Feeding and sleep patterns may be altered, rumination reduced and a stress response becomes apparent such as increased heart rate and blood indicators. Some studies show that these stress responses decrease in cows that have had several calves. There is even some evidence that cows reared in isolation are not as good mothers as cows reared with other calves. They are slow to start licking their calves and are less aggressive, demonstrating reduced motivation for social contact.

Keeping cattle in intensive environments inevitably leads to a modification of their behaviour compared with wild cattle. Behavioural needs are best determined by investigating which innate behaviours need to be performed and then, which behaviours are required to meet their physiological needs. The physiological needs include:

- absorption of adequate nutrient supplies from the gut
- perpetuation of the genotype by reproduction
- adequacy of the environment in terms of thermal and other sensory requirements.

Taking these into account, the major behavioural needs are:

- reaction to danger (flight and escape)
- ingestion
- body care (including elimination)
- motion
- exploration/territorialism
- rest
- association (including social and reproductive behaviour).

3.3.4 Interactions with humans

The permanent contact between cattle and humans makes them easier to handle, since they learn to follow the humans as their leader. Acting responsibly as the 'boss' animal brings stability to the herd, and there is evidence that cattle respond best to a person who is confident and consistent in handling them. The cattle also respond to regular communication with their keepers, particularly during periods of stress such as calving. This communication may be in the form of touching the animals, petting, stroking or scratching, particularly around the head and neck. This mimics grooming. Communication can also be verbal and visual, such as talking to and looking at cattle in their charge. Firm handling to assume dominant status combined with the caring role of the matriarchal substitute is necessary if cattle are to be contented. Modern production systems are designed for minimal labour input hence the importance of the stockperson's role in the herd is often not recognised. Investment in physical means to overcome abnormal behaviour can be reduced with greater attention to their psychological needs for adequate social bonding.

Cattle can recognise and respond to differences in human temperament that will affect their response to handling. The major types of interactions are:

- hand and arm (tactile) interaction
- vocal interaction
- holistic empathetic interactions, such as smell and other senses.

These can be pleasant (patting the back, stroking) or aversive (hitting) and performed with varying degrees of confidence. Phillips (2002) argues that some respect or fear of the stockperson may be necessary to enable cattle to be moved with ease and discourage them from attempting to force interactions with humans. It is important for a stockperson to be able to assess an animal's temperament, so that they can predict its behavioural reactions to handling and milking and modify their own behaviour accordingly.

There have been equivocal findings about the impact of handling on milk yields in dairy cows in that some researchers have found a negative relationship between aggressive handling and milk yield while others have reported no effect. Likewise, studies relating cow temperament to milk yield have been inconclusive. Farm studies have noted a change in milking personnel can lead to a change in herd milk yield, but this could be due to other changes in milking management rather than the milkers themselves. With increasing herd sizes and automation on dairy farms, such as machine feeding of total mixed rations, there may be less positive interactions between stock and humans.

Normally most contact with older cattle has neutral or negative associations, such as delivering injections, inserting intra-vaginal devices and weighing stock. These all disrupt the normal social structure within herds, bringing stock into abnormally close contact with each other and with humans and increase the risk of physical damage when stock are forced to enter races, crushes and gates in yards. Young cattle may have positive associations with humans, say, with bucket feeding, but not older stock that are often fed out of machines. Newly calved heifers have to join the rest of the milking herd so must learn to cope with being mixed with older stock and having to develop a new dominance order as well as adjusting to the new traumas associated with the twice daily routine of machine milking. The process of milking, which can relieve pressure inside the udders of high yielding cows, was thought to be the major motivation for cows to enter automatic, robotically operated milk harvesting systems, but this has not always been found to be the case. The 'promise' of extra feed is another incentive for cows to enter the milking parlour.

The herd person plays a major role in shaping the temperament of cattle in their care. Extra handling of young calves reduces their flight distance (see Chapter 4). However, such positive interactions reduce with age although regular positive contact at any age reduces the strength of the adverse reactions to later handling.

4

Cattle behaviour

This chapter discusses the details of cattle behaviour (in other words, what cattle do) such as the relative importance of the five body senses, the various ways stock communicate with each other and their keepers and behavioural problems arising from clashes with their environment.

The main points of this chapter

- Of the five senses cattle possess, sight is the most dominant. Hearing and smell also play important roles in how cows assess their environment.
- As a prey species, cattle have an inherent fear of unfamiliar objects, situations, smells, sudden movements and noises. As well they can experience fearfulness in situations where they are solitary or isolated. Understanding this is critical to managing them in a low stress manner.
- Cattle are less expressive of pain and injury than humans. Therefore, behavioural indicators of pain that cattle do express are subtle. An animal experiencing pain has compromised welfare, and consequences to their health and productivity are also likely.
- The presence of stereotypic behaviours indicate that a cow is in a compromised welfare state, and is feeling frustrated at the inability to behave naturally. In cattle, oral stereotypies, which relate to nutritional and foraging deficits, and ambulatory stereotypies, the result of restricted movement, are common.

- The intensification of cattle housing, feeding and management contributes to behavioural problems not seen in grazing animals. Frustrations lead to some cows engaging in often repetitive and pointless (stereotyped) behaviour that can be interpreted as a reflection of reduced activity, hence restricted normal behaviour, in intensively managed housing systems.
- Tongue rolling and bar chewing are two classic stereotype behaviour problems. Nymphomania, silent heats and extreme aggression towards humans are other behavioural problems in intensively managed cattle.
- Feeding vices can be attributed to boredom following a too rapid satisfying of their nutritional needs. These include dropping feed, feed throwing and water lapping.
- The behaviours of cows will change in response to the situations they are in and the handling they experience, resulting in an increased or decreased frequency of common behaviours.
- The behaviour of the cow handler has an enormous impact on cow behaviour, welfare and performance. Negative behaviours produce more fearful cows. Positive behaviour will lead to a relaxed herd of cows that are easier to handle.
- A good handler with a considerate, calm and positive attitude towards cows can lead to 20% higher milk yields over a handler with a poor attitude.

The behaviour of domestic cattle has evolved over a long time, initially in response to their domestication as discussed in the previous chapter, but more recently in response to more subtle changes in their handling, feeding and herd management as they have become more exposed to the intensive practices of modern day dairy and beef cattle farming.

4.1   The development of cow behaviour

The behaviour of cattle is determined by instinct, sensory perception and experience. Instinctual behaviours refer to those that the cow is naturally motivated to perform. Sensory behaviours are those that are the result of something heard/seen/smelt/felt in the environment.

Examples of these different types of behaviour include:

- Instinct or innate, fully developed and complete at first appearance; suckling and standing at birth, those rhythmical behaviours fundamental to the life process (such as breathing and defecation) and freezing or baulking in response to an unfamiliar noise or object. Baulking is when the animal flinches and ceases movement, that is, it is resisting what it is being led to do.

- Conditioned learning or learning by experience, which can be positive, negative or neutral; drinking milk from a bucket, mounting behaviour during copulation, eating concentrates from an out of parlour feeder, responding to a feedout wagon, milk letdown during milking as well as responding to a handler. Much of this occurs as the result of sensory perception and investigatory behaviour when cattle are first exposed to an unfamiliar environment.
- Many behaviours are a combination of these influences. Mounting behaviour during copulation is a good example of this, with the novice bull being instinctually driven to attempt mounting, but the technique of mounting improving with experience.

Breeding programs to select for product-specific livestock can alter stock's physical and possibly behavioural attributes. For example breeding beef cattle for high lean meat content, such as producing 'double muscled' stock, can adversely impact on the natural delivery of calves during parturition, while selecting for rapid growth can lead to genetic leg disorders. With regard to dairy stock, selection for high milk production has reduced the meat producing attributes of their offspring, while the high nutrient demands for milk production often leads to lactation anoestrus (or delays in oestral cycling in newly calved cows). Furthermore, the oestrus cycle can be manipulated artificially through exogenous hormone implants.

Genetic selection for tameness has continued long after animals have been domesticated due to increased culling rates of stock that are difficult to handle. But the increased mechanisation of animal farming has shifted the target for artificial selection towards efficiency of production rather than handling ease. Selection of dairy stock for more intensive production may have produced more nervous and aggressive animals making them more difficult to handle.

Such intensive breeding programs can reduce the genetic variability within a species with unexpected consequences. For example, Phillips (2002) argues that the recent outbreak of 'mad cow disease' in the UK could be partly attributed to the increased susceptibility to the disease due to the lack of genetic diversity in the country's population of Friesian dairy cows, as a result of intense selection for high cow performance. Such are the unpredictable impacts on cattle survivability. This was then impaired animal welfare brought about by too much emphasis on economic performance.

Vices develop, such as tongue rolling as a result of the thwarting of natural behaviours and such abnormal behaviour appears to be under genetic control (see the following section). It may in fact be possible to breed stock that do not perform these abnormal behaviours and this could result in improving their welfare status because they do not find the environment as frustrating. However, some of the abnormal behaviours noted may provide relief from frustration and thereby improve the animal's welfare. The fact that these behaviours exist in the first place, however, are indicative of a welfare issue that needs to be addressed. The behaviour of domesticated stock seems to be more flexible than their wild ancestors and could include the capacity to develop such stereotypies as part of their coping mechanisms in our modern day, and often less animal friendly, production systems.

Cattle are social animals. Forming a herd reduces the risk of predation by leaving large areas of grazing land open and reducing the chance of a predator seeing an individual animal or picking up its trail. In addition, predation is reduced by the rapid flight of large numbers of animals in random directions thereby confusing the predator. Also the opportunity of members of a herd learning survival tactics is increased through social facilitation.

Cattle are animals that fear novelty but become accepting of a routine. They have good memories and stock with previous experience of gentle handling will be easier to deal with than stock with a history of rough handling. A better understanding of natural behaviour will facilitate handling. Being prey animals, fear motivates them to be constantly vigilant in order to escape from predators. When cattle become agitated during handling, they are motivated by fear. Calm animals are then easier to handle. Fearful animals stick together making handling more difficult. If cattle become frightened, it can take 20 min for them to calm down.

Although cattle are creatures of habit, gentle dairy cows can easily be prompted into movement that is dangerous to both the animal and handler by the use of unnecessary severe methods of handling (such as shouting and electric prods) and restraint. Attempts to force an animal to do something it does not want to do often end in failure and can cause the animal to become confused, disorientated, frightened or upset. Handling cattle requires them to be 'outsmarted' rather than be 'outfought' and they should be 'outwaited' rather than hurried. Most tests of will between the handler and the cows are won by the cow.

Recent management practices that have improved comfort and wellbeing in dairy cows include:

- raising calves in comfortable pens or shelters, including contact with other calves
- providing exercise before calving
- grooving or roughening polished, smooth concrete flooring to prevent slipping
- making use of pasture or earthen exercise lots and removing slatted floors
- eliminating stray voltage.

When cows ruminate, they appear relaxed with their head down and their eyelids lowered. Resting cows prefer to lie on their chest, facing slightly uphill. Also, through cud chewing as well as mutual and self-grooming, aggression is reduced and there is little or no boredom.

Females of dairy breeds on heat are reputed to mount more than those of beef breeds. It has been argued that this is the result of greater selection for this trait in systems where males are largely or completely absent (Chenoweth and Landaeta-Hernandez 1998). The widespread use of artificial insemination in dairy herds may have led to unplanned selection for cows showing overt oestrus behaviour because those showing weak signs of oestrus would be less easily identified and therefore inseminated.

In feral cattle, herd social organisation usually takes the form of groups of mothers and offspring, and bachelor groups of bulls grazing separately. These groupings are related to the dominance of the stock within each one and so are often called social dominance groups. Dominant bulls join the cow herd when there are oestrous cows, which is their signal for mounting behaviour. In domesticated cattle these social dominance groups are replaced by groups of cows and growing cattle, usually divided into similar age and single sex groups after about 6 months of age. Bulls kept for reproduction may be solitary confined for much of their life, or they may run with the herd of cows or even be rotated between herds. These changes in social structure from the natural groupings and the intensive husbandry methods used, increase social tension. With growing male cattle or bulls, the stresses of close confinement may make them difficult to manage safely without danger to the stockperson, with castration used to improve their temperament by reducing aggression.

As cattle handlers, it is important to understand both innate behaviours of cattle and how our actions can modify their responses. This chapter aims to outline both of these fundamental principles that have such an important impact on how cattle behave.

4.2   The five senses

4.2.1   Vision

Vision is the dominant sense in cattle and is responsible for about half of the sensory information they receive from their surroundings. Cattle have a 330° vision, of this visual area, they have binocular vision for a limited area in front of them. This is where they will have the clearest vision and ability to judge depth or distance. In order to get the best possible vision, cattle will lower their head and face the stimulus of interest front on.

The rest of their visual field is monocular. This large monocular area is very good for detecting predators, but they cannot judge distance here well. Because of this poorer depth perception here, it is best to approach a cow from the side, but moving at a slow pace. This will not spook the cow and allow you to approach more closely than front on.

The remaining area around the cow is referred to as the blind spot. This is the area directly behind the cow's tail. If you approach the cow from her blind spot she will not know you are there. Suddenly moving into or out of this position can upset the animal and lead to flighty and unpredictable behaviour.

Cattle are less able to discriminate objects that differ in light intensity and cannot see red colours as well as humans. This increases their colour contrast, making shadows look more extreme compared to how we perceive them. Paired with limited depth perception, a block of shadow can look like a hole in the ground to cattle. Shadows, very bright light and sparkling reflections will distract or slow down cattle investigating their surroundings, often upsetting the smooth flow of cows in a laneway. Cattle are also motivated to move from areas of low light to well lit areas. Conversely, they will avoid moving from well lit to dark areas.

Taking cattle's visual sense into consideration is very important when trying to move them. In both free moving and tethered cattle, moving them can be much easier if lighting is even, the area free of distracting and unfamiliar objects, and you don't make sudden, significant movements.

4.2.2 Hearing

Cattle are very sensitive to high frequency sounds and have a wider range of hearing than humans (a human's auditory range is from 64 to 23 000 Hz, cattle's from 23 to 35 000 Hz). Despite having a greater range of auditory detection than people, cattle have greater difficulty in locating the origin of sounds and will use their sight to assist them determine the source. High pitched noises such as whistling are also unpleasant to cows. Intermittent sounds such as clanging of metal (e.g. gates), shouting and whistling can be particularly stressful, especially if they are sudden and at a loud volume.

4.2.3 Smell

Due to their evolution as prey animals, cattle have a very acute sense of smell. Cattle select their feed on the basis of smell and can detect odours many kilometres away. They will avoid places containing urine from stressed animals, and for this reason may be reluctant to enter places where cattle have been previously handled such as raceways and cattle crushes. They dislike the smells of dung and saliva, so when housed, their feeding area needs to be kept clean and smell fresh, not contaminated with dung, saliva or exudate from other cows' noses. Herd hierarchy is strongly linked to smell, as shown by studies where the social order among cows was unaltered by blindfolding them.

As well as a sensitive nose, they have an additional olfactory sensitive organ, called the vomeronasal organ, on the roof of their mouth. The reception of odours by this organ is used for the reinforcement and maintenance of sexual interest. When seeking and finding a suitable cow on heat, this is characterised by the 'flehman expression' in mating bulls, in which the head is directed upwards with the mouth ajar, the tongue flat and the upper lips curled back. This is thought to aid odour sampling by allowing air to contact the roof of the mouth during inhalation. Bulls appear to increase their olfactory behaviour about four days before cows show signs of oestrus.

The production and detection of pheromones is another way cattle seek out suitable stock for mating. For this reason, cows on heat spend much time sniffing and licking the anal and vaginal areas of other cows. Other pheromones convey fear. Cattle respond to pheromones produced in fearful situations by increasing their own physiological stress response and fear behaviours. Cattle are also sensitive to the odours of potential predators, like dogs, spending more time sniffing the air and in cautious movement. In comparison to humans, cattle are able to detect much smaller differences in odour concentration.

4.2.4 Taste

There are four primary tastes identifiable in cattle. These are:

- sweetness (associated with energy supply)
- saltiness (associated with electrolyte balance)
- bitterness (assists to avoid toxins and tannins that reduce the nutritive value of plants)
- acidity (linked to pH balance).

The taste receptors are located in specific areas of the tongue, with differences between cattle and humans in their taste discrimination, sensitivity and location on the tongue. Cattle have two to three times as many taste buds as humans, and so are more sensitive to tastes. Cattle can be apprehensive when it comes to eating novel food – feed with unfamiliar tastes and smells. For example, they need artificial sweeteners to mask bitter tastes such as zinc in water.

4.2.5 Touch

Skin receptors are used to detect pressure, movement, temperature and some damaging pathological conditions such as inflammation. Humans have increased sensitivity in their fingertips whereas cattle often use their extended mouth as a sampling tool in exploratory situations.

Cattle perceive extreme ambient temperatures, relative humidities and/or wind speed through thermoreceptors, skin dryness (particularly in the throat and nasal passages) and mechanoreceptors. They learn their comfort or thermoneutral zones, above and below which they must use physiological processes to sustain their core body temperatures. They then modify their behaviour accordingly, such as seeking cooler locations during hot weather to find more favourable microclimates. As the lower critical temperature of adult cows is −23°C, they are rarely affected by cold stress. Heat stress is a common problem, at 21°C cattle increase their respiration rate, and at 25°C, above which they reduce feed intake to reduce metabolic heat production from rumen fermentation. Breed differences also influence the susceptibility of cattle to heat loads. Factors like higher metabolic rate, greater amounts of body fat and thicker coats all increase the likelihood of cattle suffering from heat stress. These breed differences are important considerations in the tropics.

Cattle can readily detect low-level electric current, which often exists in milking parlours where wet conditions and connection of machinery to their udders make cattle prone to stray voltage. As the resistance provided by humans is two to 10 times greater (depending on footwear), the level of current that will disturb cows is much lower than it is for humans.

4.3 Behavioural indicators of poor welfare

The intensification of cattle housing and dairy cattle management contributes to behavioural problems not seen in grazing animals. Restriction of normal behaviours due to the production systems imposed on them are most frequently at the root of behavioural problems in cattle. Cattle, as with other domesticated species, have fewer behavioural problems when left in their natural environment. Therefore, there is a concern that intensive management has resulted in the decline of the animal's wellbeing. In some cases, the way that stock behave is the only clue that discomfort and distress are present. This can be even more subtle with tethered animals.

4.3.1 Pain and its detection

While pain detection is related to touch, we have included it here in a separate category because it is of major importance to cattle welfare.

Cattle have similar mechanisms for sensing pain as humans do, with responses increasing with the magnitude and duration of the stimuli. Situations cattle are in can influence their responsiveness to pain. Pain is reduced in cattle kept with herd mates (known as conspecifics) and greater when cows are isolated. Being aware of this factor when conducting any painful husbandry practices is important.

Cattle are less expressive of pain and injury than humans. This is an evolved mechanism, with it being disadvantageous for prey animals to express pain or weakness, as weakness makes them an easier target for predators (Phillips 2002). Therefore, the behavioural indicators of pain that cattle do express are subtle. An animal experiencing pain has compromised welfare, and consequences to their health and productivity are also likely.

Common behavioural indicators are as follows:

- Abnormal stance and gait. Stances indicating pain may include a tucked abdomen and tail, hunched back or standing still for extended periods of time. Abnormal gait can include unusual walking patterns (e.g. walking backwards), or uneven weight bearing, as seen when a cow is suffering from lameness.
- Unusual resting behaviours. Lying with legs in an unusual position and a hesitation to rise when lying may indicate pain. Dog sitting may occur when

the animal is trying to keep the painful area off the ground while trying to rest (see Figure 4.4).

- Vocalisations. These can act as a warning to other cattle to avoid a painful situation, or an involuntary response to painful stimuli. Anecdotal evidence suggests that Asian cattle vocalise less than Western breeds.
- Kicking and tail swishing. Both may be performed in response to acute pain and may be directed towards the painful stimulus.
- Very subtle indicators. These can include teeth grinding, reduced food intake and an absence of rumination.

Some of the above examples are indicative of specific painful experiences, while others are more general. In many situations of compromise, the provision of pain relief will improve the animal's welfare and recovery.

4.3.2   Fear and its implications

Fear is the response to a real or perceived threat and serves to protect the animal from danger. As they have evolved as prey animals, cows are naturally reactive or fearful in several different situations, including a fear of novelty. As a result cattle can find unfamiliar objects, situations and smells and sudden movements and noises frightening. This is exacerbated when they are solitary or isolated. It is for this reason that gentle handling, repeated exposure to situations or environments and a consistent routine can help to create calm animals. Improved cow movement and milk yield are measurable benefits arising from 'cow friendly' facility design and stock handling practices.

In the same way that cows can learn to become relaxed if they are treated well and exposed to stimuli in a consistent, calm way, they can also learn to fear an environment, situation or handler. Below are examples of situations that commonly elicit fear in cattle. Repeated exposure to these sorts of events will result in cattle displaying fear in anticipation of a situation. As a result, they will be more flighty and difficult to handle. With gentle handling and routine, cows will be easier to move, easier to milk, and will let down more milk.

Examples of fear-eliciting situations are as listed by Klindworth *et al.* (2003):

- Sudden movements or noises are very threatening to cows. Moving and handling animals in a calm, quiet way can significantly reduce fear. Associated fear behaviours (such as startling, baulking, fleeing) can result when cattle interpret some relatively common situations as threats, such as heights, sudden movement, sudden noises, threatening or aggressive actions, prolonged eye contact and large or towering objects. These evolutionary threats can be minimised through good dairy and shed design and thoughtful stock handling.
- Cows can find novelty fearful, and are generally afraid of sudden changes to facilities and routines. Keeping environmental features such as lighting, floor

surfaces or levels, and fences or wall types as consistent as possible will help to reduce fear. If cows become fearful in a new situation, try and allow them some time to familiarise themselves with the new environment before introducing further changes or other stressful procedures. Rushing cows when they are slow because of novelty (and so are fearful) will exacerbate the issue.

- Cows will fear humans if handled poorly and they associate this poor handling with the place where it occurred. Using the cows' natural behaviour to guide handling and other interactions will minimise fear responses.
- Fear can make handling and milking harder, more time consuming and more dangerous. It can also delay milk letdown (for up to 20 min) and reduce milk yields (by up to 20%).
- Fear responses during movement make cows more prone to slipping, falling and injuries (e.g. pelvic and hip injuries due to falling, hoof injuries during slipping leading to lameness, for example) and compromise their welfare.

Improved cow movement and milk yield are measurable benefits arising from 'cow friendly' facility design and stock handling practices.

4.3.3   Descriptors of cow behaviour

A wide variety of terms can be used to describe cow behaviour, such as the 20 used by Welfare Quality (2009) in their welfare assessment protocols. These are listed below in decreasing order of positive emotional state:

Happy, content, positively occupied, friendly, relaxed, calm, active, sociable, playful, lively, inquisitive, uneasy, bored, indifferent, fearful, apathetic, frustrated, agitated, distressed, irritable.

When describing antagonistic behaviours, Welfare Quality (2009) use the following descriptors:

- *head butting*; which occurs with physical contact where one animal is butting, hitting, thrusting, striking or pushing the other animal with forehead, horns or horn base with a forceful movement; the receiver does not give up its present position
- *displacement*; which is physical contact where one animal is forcing the other animal to give up its position
- *chasing*; where one animal makes another animal move
- *fighting*; where two animals push their heads against each other while planting their feet on the ground with both exerting force against each other
- *chasing-up*; where one animal uses physical contact against a lying animal to make it rise.

4.3.4   Stereotypic behaviours

Stereotypic behaviour is a term applied to repeated sequences of a behaviour that has no apparent purpose or benefit and is caused by the frustration of natural behaviour patterns or repeated attempts to deal with some problem (Mason and Rushen 2006). These are behaviours that have replaced natural ones that have been repressed by the artificial conditions of management. Compared to non-ruminant species such as poultry, cattle generally display fewer stereotypic behaviours when kept intensively. The more restrictive the management, the higher the frequency of their occurrence. Different species perform different stereotypies, and the type of stereotypic behaviour usually relates to the root cause. In cattle, these are usually oral stereotypies, which relate to nutritional and foraging deficits. Ambulatory stereotypies, the result of restricted movement, are also common. Tongue playing or rolling, bar biting, prepuce or scrotum biting and urine drinking are behaviours commonly referred to as stereotypies in cattle.

Oral stereotypies are common in cattle when kept intensively because they no longer perform the long amounts of grazing and ruminating that they would when on pasture, which accounts for more than 9 h of their time budget naturally (Mason and Rushen 2006). With tongue rolling or tongue playing, the animal curls and uncurls the tongue inside or outside their mouth. After that, partial swallowing of the tongue and gulping of air may take place. In addition to this, object licking and bar biting are common. Bar biting consists of clamping the jaws around a bar and moving the head back and forth while chewing on the bar.

Along with restricted grazing, ambulatory stereotypic behaviours develop as a result of tethering. Tethered cattle show pacing and swaying behaviours, suggesting frustrations with an inability to move. Swaying is particularly prevalent and has been reported in up to 20% of the tethered herd (Blaszak 2011).

Research has shown that a combination of oral and ambulatory stereotypies have been found to occur in previously grazed cows that were then continuously tethered over many months (Albright and Arave 1997). These behaviours were linked to frustration resulting from a greatly reduced opportunity for activity (walking) along with reduced psychological and physiological contacts and the manipulation and processing of their feed. Environmental stimulation in the form of 1 h of exercise (e.g. loose in a pen area) each day can reduce incidences of bar biting in tethered cows, while tongue rolling ceases altogether following the transfer from tethering to loose housing or grazing. The provision of straw or hay, which increases chewing and ruminating time, is recommended to combat this.

Such oral manipulation, tongue playing and non-nutritive sucking is also very apparent in veal calves that are individually stalled and only fed milk and concentrates. Feeding long hay reduces such abnormal behaviour in stall fed calves while they are absent altogether in calves suckled by their dams and grazed for 6 h per day (Albright and Arave 1997). Housing calves in pairs or small groups will also reduce the incidences of stereotypical behaviour, and address their other behavioural needs (see Chapter 3).

Grandin and Deesing (1998) considered tongue rolling to be a relatively new abnormal behaviour and mainly apparent in intensively managed (generally lofted)

Friesian beef steers and dairy heifers and cows. They also considered it may need to be performed to satisfy their instinct of prehension of forage plants during grazing as it is seen most frequently immediately before and after feeding. As well as rolling their tongues with their mouths open, these cattle excessively lick every surface in the feedlot pen, such as fences and gates. Grandin and Deesing (1998) attributed this phenomenon to overselection for high levels of milk production in Friesians. In order for Friesian steers to maintain such high growth rates, or for Friesian cows to produce large volumes of milk, they must consume large quantities of feed, for which they have been genetically selected for large appetites. This pointless licking of fences and gates might be a precursor to more serious problems if genetic selection for the highest production is continued. These authors also pointed out that Friesian steers on high grain rations tended to have more bloat than beef steers on similar rations. In addition to bloat, they reported grain-fed Friesian steers to have higher levels of sudden death than beef cattle. Grandin and Deesing (1998) then interpreted these observations as a caution in that intensive genetic selection programs for high performance may need to be more seriously considered in the light of these ongoing concerns about animal welfare.

In addition to tongue rolling, prepuce sucking and urine drinking are frequently observed in intensively managed fattening bulls. In one study, incidence of these behaviours were very high for urine drinking (53%), sucking and licking and biting of ears (44%), sucking and licking of the prepuce or scrotum and tongue rolling (38%) and licking and biting of tails (1%). Such high incidences of abnormal behaviour were associated with too little space per animal, rations with no dry forage and difficult access to water. Despite being offered sufficient feed of high quality and adequate drinking water, tongue rolling is still apparent, even in well-managed dairy farms in SE Asia.

The presence of these stereotypic behaviours indicate that a cow is in a compromised welfare state, and is feeling frustrated at the inability to perform natural behaviours. As indicated in the examples above, simple modifications to the animal's environment will reduce these behaviours and improve the animal's welfare.

4.4   Animal movement
4.4.1   Flight zone and point of balance
The flight zone is the area around an animal that if penetrated will cause the animal to move or flee. It specifically relates to stimuli that the animal considers to be threatening, and it extends around the whole animal. Entering the flight zone will cause the animal to move, as it aims to re-establish a safe distance between itself and the perceived threat. Because the animal's senses are concentrated towards the reception of signals from the front, the flight distance is greater in

front of than behind the animal. The flight zones of cows differ between individuals, and are influenced by things like environment, temperament, age and previous experience. The flight zone of a cow will also change depending on the situation they are in. Novel and stressful situations will increase the flight zone of the animal, as will unfamiliar people. As they become habituated or relaxed in a situation, the flight zone will reduce. The pace at which you enter the flight zone will also influence the cow's behaviour. Rapidly moving into the flight zone will stimulate the flight response of cattle, whereas gentle movement will still cause the animal to move away, but it will do so more slowly. Figures 4.1, 4.2 and 4.3 provide a graphical depiction of the flight zone and point of balance.

Generally, the flight zone of loose housed cattle in large-scale commercial dairy herds is 3 to 5 m, although it could be smaller on smallholder farms where the stock are handled more frequently. Permanently tethering milking cows is also likely to reduce their flight zone because of their more frequent contact with people, and the animal knowing that it cannot move away. In intensive systems, the flight distance is by necessity reduced, compared with, for example, an open range. Dairy cattle have a smaller flight distance than beef cattle. This would have resulted from more frequent handling and interaction with people, on dairy farms compared to beef farms, and genetic selection for closer flight zones during the

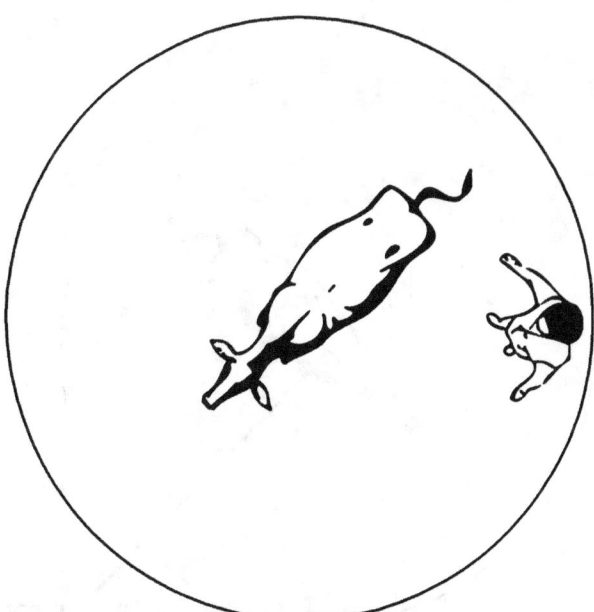

Figure 4.1: Flight zone: the flight zone of a cow is an invisible boundary around the animal and is the minimum distance that the animal feels safe from you. Moving into the flight zone will cause the animal to move as it tries to re-establish this safe distance.

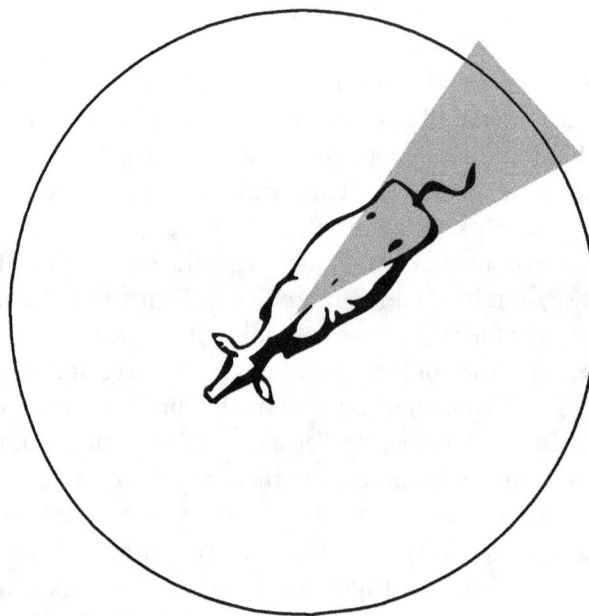

Figure 4.2: Blind spot: the cow cannot see you if you are in her blind spot. Sudden movement in this area will cause her to startle.

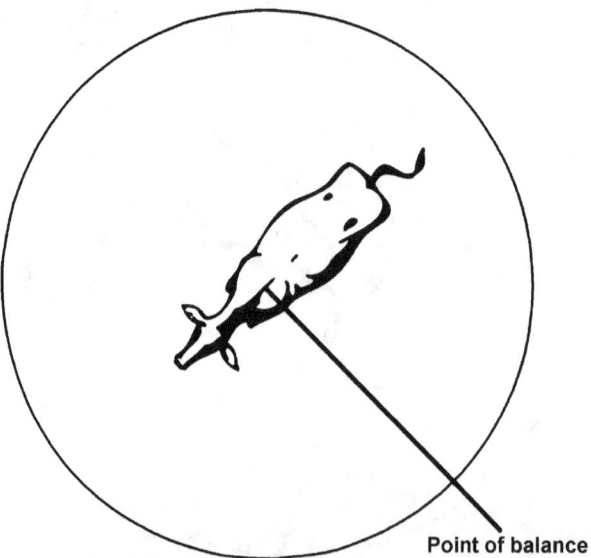

Point of balance

Figure 4.3: Point of balance: moving into an animal's flight zone in front of this point of balance (in front of the shoulder), will cause the cow to move backwards. Moving into an animal's flight zone from behind this point of balance will cause the cow to move forwards.

domestic evolution of dairy cattle. In the same way that fearfulness can either increase or decrease with experience, the flight zone will depend on the animal's history. Cows that have positive handling experiences will have a smaller flight zone than those with negative experiences.

4.4.2   Individual animal movement

In cattle, this flight zone can be used successfully to aid animal movement. Entering the flight zone will encourage the cow to move, to re-establish it. The direction and posture by which you move into the flight zone will influence how the animal moves. The handler's position and direction of approach in relation to the cow's 'point of balance' determines the direction the cow will move in. The point of balance is an imaginary line through the animal's shoulder.

If you enter the flight zone from in front of the cow (in front of the point of balance) it will cause her to move backwards. Entering from behind the shoulder (behind the point of balance) will cause her to move forwards.

Animals tethered by the nose or halter are conditioned to move in response to leading. They are prompted to move by the forward movement of the handler, effectively the opposite to the point of balance and flight zone described above. When moving a tethered animal it is important to keep in mind stimuli that will cause an animal to baulk. Loud noises, unfamiliar sounds and sights, will all cause an animal to stop moving. Pulling too hard on the tether can be both painful to the animal and futile for you. Avoiding these fear-inducing situations or slowly and calmly leading cows through this area is a better option. A cow that is comfortable with its environment and handler should move easily when required.

4.4.3   Herd movement

When untethered, the forced movement of cattle initially creates an order unrelated to dominance, because the dominant animals are interspersed throughout the herd. However, subordinate cattle gradually move to the front on the herd and the most dominant animals stay in the middle, leading the herd by 'pushing' rather than 'pulling'. There is also a reluctance to be at the back of the mob, as these animals are the most exposed and closest to the human (or predator) driving them.

When moving the herd, keep in mind that cattle will naturally group and move together; movement of other cows triggers the next cows to move. The pace at which you push the herd will influence the pace of their movement. A slow, consistent pace is best as this ensures safe movement, reducing the risks of injury and lameness, or of causing panic in the herd.

Calm people have calm cows and calm cows give more milk and have fewer problems such as hoof conditions. It is important to let cows move at their own pace because hurrying them up achieves little else other than making the last few cows in a group nervous. Cows generally walk in some order of rank and do not overtake each other. When they are calm, they keep their heads down so they can see where they are placing their feet. They only lift their heads when they become nervous. Since cows are creatures of habit, they like to learn exactly what is happening, what they have to do and when. So it is important to have patience to allow routines to develop, then rigidly stick to these routines. A group of cows moves like a flowing stream, so to prevent this stream from being interrupted, it is important to avoid obstacles, passageways with dead ends and things that make cows feel afraid.

4.5   Social behaviours

Cattle are social animals and have evolved to live in herds in a strategy to reduce the risk of predation. Grazing in open areas increases the risk of predation, and group living increases the likelihood of predator detection to compensate. Another protective element of herds – the rapid flight or stampede of large numbers of animals – confuses predators during attack. The opportunity of members of a herd learning survival tactics is also increased through social facilitation.

Importantly, this evolution of social behaviour means that isolation is particularly stressful to cattle. Isolation can cause animals to be distressed and panic, increasing the likelihood of injury to both the individual and handler. The effect of isolation is additive or compounding, with animals being more stressed during husbandry procedures when isolated. Therefore, it is always best to keep several animals together during activities like veterinary treatment, artificial insemination or movement from one place to another.

4.5.1   Visual communication

Visual signs are one of the main methods used by cattle to communicate, particularly to indicate aggressive and reproductive states (discussed below). For tethered animals, the ability to express these methods of communication are limited, as a result, they will be more subtle than those in free moving cows.

The signals of aggression displayed by bulls take the form of lowering of the head, drawing the chin towards the body and inclining the horns to the opponent, signalling their intention to charge by pawing the ground. In cows, the threat is less forceful and generally involves head swinging for aggressive displays and turning away as a submissive signal. The ability of tethered cattle to display submissive signals to dominant animals will be limited, and as a result, aggressive interactions should be monitored carefully, and cows moved if aggressive behaviours continue.

The tail is an important signalling device in cattle. The tail will usually be held horizontal during defecation and urination. If, together with the head, it is elevated, this often indicates an exploratory situation to investigate the source of some stimulus. Tails are also elevated during oestrus display, fighting, threats, greetings, suckling and homosexual activities in both males and females. Conversely when the tail is held between the legs, this indicates the animal is cold or frightened or fearful. Lateral movements of the tail are often used for fly removal, but can be a response to more general cutaneous irritations such as rubbing or stimulation such as of vulva or penis during sexual behaviour. Tail wagging is also common when cattle are being irritated. Cows will wag their tail as a threat if they are about to kick. Tail wagging can also be performed in response to painful stimuli.

Facial expressions are of less importance because the facial musculature is less well developed than in other species, and the distance between animals would often preclude the use of facial gestures as signals. Some obvious signals are present, however. The flehman response has already been discussed in relation to oestrus. Situations causing arousal (surprise, alarm, distress) will cause an increase in the size of the white of the eye surrounding the pupil. Conversely, cattle often perform routine behaviours, such as eating, ruminating or lying with their eyes half closed, which may be an indication of relaxation. Ear movement may also be involved in expressive behaviour, as they are in sheep, but this is yet to be researched. Ear postures will change in response to auditory signals, allowing the cow to locate the direction of a sound.

Grooming is primarily a body care activity but it has additional benefits. Cattle groom each other (allogrooming), usually the head and neck region of animals that are of similar or slightly subordinate positions in the dominance order. They may groom each other to maintain dominance position, to reinforce family bonds and those between adult cattle. Abilities to allogroom and reinforce bonds is also limited in tethered animals. Providing the opportunity for animals to interact and perform these behaviours is important.

4.5.2 Vocal communication

Vocal communication is used in recognition, eliciting contact as well as greetings, threats and fear display. Certain types of calls are associated with specific behaviours or emotional states. With calves, the calls during isolation are of lower frequency and carry further than during branding, perhaps suggesting greater stress. As an animal becomes more excited or distressed, the duration, volume and pitch of the calls increase. Vocalisations have been categorised and calls fall into five 'main syllables' based on the mouth, tongue and nasal placement and the speed of air leaving the throat (Phillips 2002). Other classifications use amplitude, pitch, tonality and length to interpret the message of different calls. Calls change as the animal ages, and bulls tend to vocalise more than cows and steers.

The frequency of vocalisations can be used as an indicator of cattle welfare in abattoirs and during handling. Vocalisations can also indicate pain. However, as yet, no specific meaning has been attributed to different calls.

4.5.3 Reproductive behaviour

Cows indicate reproductive receptivity by homosexual mounting, where the cow exhibiting the standing reflex is receptive, not necessarily the mounting cow. Mounting cows, although not necessarily receptive, are usually approaching receptivity so their activity indicates they may benefit from the presence of a bull. In herds where the bull is removed from the herd, such homosexual mounting is of great benefit to the stockperson to indicate the right time to bring in a bull or to use artificial insemination. Females of dairy breeds on heat are reputed to mount more than those of beef breeds. It has been argued that this is the result of greater selection for this trait in systems where males are largely or completely absent (Chenoweth and Landaeta-Hernandez 1998). The widespread use of artificial insemination in dairy herds may have led to unplanned selection for cows showing overt oestrus behaviour because those showing weak signs of oestrus would be less easily identified and so inseminated.

In confinement, there are about 14 different behavioural sexual activities, and cow-to-cow mounting is the most accurate sign that the time is right for insemination or taking the cow to the bull. Reasons for failed visual detection of oestrus include inappropriate flooring, with bulls and cows being unwilling to mount when on slippery, unsteady surfaces and oestrus behaviours being performed overnight and therefore go unobserved. Despite the fact that the senior author has been told by numerous farmers in different Asian countries that they can detect cows on heat as well as a bull can, visual oestrus detection is only about 50% successful in most herds.

Mounting behaviour is also not possible to be observed in tie stall housing. For good oestrus detection, cows should be allowed access to a dirt exercise yard once or twice daily for a minimum of 1 h each time.

4.5.4 Cow–calf bonding

Cow–calf bonding is both a learnt and innate behaviour. The bond is created at a time when the calf is naturally drawn to the dam by wanting to suckle and the chances of other bonds developing during this period of primary socialisation are small. Grooming during and after suckling preserves the imprinting bond, but sight, smell and vocal communications are important for reunion of the calf and dam. This bond, and in particular suckling, maintains the post partum anoestrus in cows for about 8 weeks to prevent early rebreeding.

Intensely selected dairy breeds show weak cow–calf bonding, probably because of the routine practice of early separation of cow and calf. Artificial rearing has little effect on the calf's temperament and cross fostering is also easy.

4.5.5 Communicating with the calf

Calves have many, often quite subtle, ways to communicate their feelings to humans. Staff should learn to closely observe and interpret changes in both calf appearance and their normal behaviour, which may be symptomatic of stress or illness. This topic has been covered in detail in a previous book written by the senior author and the reader is referred to Chapter 12 on Moran (2012b) for further details.

4.5.6 Social dynamics in free moving herds

Much of this section is specific to untethered, free moving dairy systems. As farms expand in herd size, these types of systems are likely to become more common. Creating awareness of these issues beforehand will allow expanding production systems to address them before they arise.

In wild cattle, herd social organisation usually takes the form of groups of mothers and offspring, and bachelor groups of bulls grazing separately. These groupings are related to the dominance of the stock within each one, and so are often called social dominance groups. Dominant bulls can join the cow herd when there are cows displaying oestrus (or mounting behaviour). Depending on farm management systems, these social dominance groups are replaced by groups of cows and growing cattle, usually divided into similar age and single sex groups after about 6 months of age. In these extensive herds, bulls kept for reproduction may be solitarily confined for much of their life. These changes in social structure from the natural groupings and the intensive husbandry methods used can increase social tension. With growing male cattle or bulls, the stresses of close confinement may make them difficult to manage safely without danger to the stockperson. This is one of the main reasons castration is performed, to improve their temperament by reducing aggression.

Within the herd, there is a dominance hierarchy. The hierarchy usually depends on the temperament of the animal, her age and her size. Aggressive (or agonistic) behaviours are one of the ways these hierarchies are established, and introducing new animals into the herd will likely lead to hierarchies needing to be re-established. It is important to give cattle enough space so subordinate individuals can avoid confrontation.

Herd size

Herd size will influence the social dynamics. Herd sizes and space allowances are also not often a point of consideration on typical SHD farms in the tropics, often limited by land availability and affordability as well as knowledge. However, as smallholders become more experienced and competent, they may have greater opportunities to increase their farm and herd size. For example, there is also increasing interest in SHD farmers to combine their smaller herds in the one shed or use shared facilities, hence handling large numbers of stock may be of relevance; these cow colonies are further discussed in Section 9.2.3 in Chapter 9.

In untethered systems, as herd size increases, the frequency of agonistic interactions increases as the result of increased competition for resources. Albright and Arave (1997) noted that the provision of 3.5 m of walking space per cow and at least one feeding space and one cubicle per cow could significantly reduce social stress, highlighting the importance of resource allocation in a changing herd. In addition to this, as the size of the herd increases, individual members have difficulty in remembering the social status of other members, leading to prolonged dominance-related aggression. In young calves where no dominance order has been formed, group size has little effect on the frequency of agonistic encounters (Albright and Arave 1997).

Mixing

When cattle groups are mixed, a new dominance structure is created, usually within 24 to 72 h, depending on the degree of change in the group. Minor changes result in a doubling of aggression activity for about 24 h. Changes in the group structure may sometimes cause sufficient disruption to actually reduce feed intake and hence milk production. However, this can be quite variable, varying from 19% to zero reduced milk yields in eight different studies (Phillips 2002).

4.6   Cattle–human interactions

4.6.1   Temperament

A cow's temperament is one of the key aspects of their personality in relation to their reaction to humans. It relates to fearfulness or reaction to fearful stimuli rather than aggression, which reflects the position in the dominance order. An animal's temperament relates strongly to previous handling experiences (positive or negative) and handling frequency. There are also genetic differences, with variety between breeds and between sires within breeds. For example, Friesian cattle are more sensitive to sound and touch in auctions than beef breeds.

Subjective scoring systems describing temperament as placid, docile, nervous or lively, correlate well with more objective measures of heart rate and breathing rate. Docile cows tend to produce more milk, this may be related to being more calm during milking and therefore having greater milk letdown. Some cattle react strongly to human presence, and can remember aversive handlers in the milking parlour thus leading to reduced milk production and poorer reproductive performance.

Cattle usually improve their temperament and become less fearful with age, as this is associated with habituation, with the animal becoming more familiar with handling procedures and the environment.

It is likely that handling experiences as a calf influence temperament, as bad handling during this critical period will render an animal nervous and hypersensitive to stress. Therefore, it is beneficial to positively condition calves to handling from an early age. Exposing calves to novel, but positive experiences in early life will lead to a cow better habituated to novelty and more docile towards people.

4.6.2 Behaviour of the cow handler

The cow handler has an enormous impact, and can be considered the most important factor influencing cow behaviour, welfare and performance. Negative behaviours, such as hitting, slapping, tail twisting, quick and sudden actions and shouting, produce more fearful cows. Once humans enter the flight zones of entrapped, fearful stock, their behaviours can become even more unpredictable. Even less obvious negative behaviours, such as mild slaps and pushes, can lead to heightened levels of fear of people. Poor treatment of cattle will also initiate a continual cycle of increasing fear and poor behaviour in the herd. Negative human behaviours will make cattle more fearful and harder to handle, which then increases the incidences of hitting, pushing, yelling and other negative behaviours in the handler. Positive interactions and handler behaviours include slow and gentle movements, rubbing or resting a hand on the cow's back or flank, and gentle vocal communication at an even volume, will lead to a relaxed herd of cows, generating easier handling and better herd health and performance.

To improve stockpersonship we need to pay attention to the level of job satisfaction of the people who care and handle the stock. To reduce rough handling, we need to understand the situation in which people become rough with animals. Educating stockpeople on the best ways to handle cattle will help improve cow movement and encourage positive human behaviour. Poorly designed facilities can make cattle more difficult to move, leading to frustrations in the staff. Correcting for this where possible and providing low-stress handling techniques to staff can help to reduce staff frustration. Other routine tasks such as hoof trimming are essential for the good welfare of stock but are often rated as unpleasant by the staff. Designing better equipment and facilities for such tasks may result in them being carried out more often and more effectively.

Adopting strategies to behave positively towards cows is the key to reducing fear of humans in cows and this can be best achieved by developing good handling practices and routines, such as:

- Keep herd handling routines (milking, veterinary treatments) consistent and calm
- Allow time for cows to learn any change in routine
- Use positive interactions such as a stroke or a rub or resting the hand on the cow's back
- Scratch the cow or give her feed as a reward after a bad experience
- Use slow and deliberate movement and talking

- Reduce excessive noise, such as banging gates and shouting
- Avoid staring at a cow directly for long periods
- Move stock by working at the edge of their flight zone
- Avoid painful procedures in the milking parlour
- Move cattle as a group rather than individually
- Use rewards to mask or minimise unpleasant experiences such as restraint or vaccination.

Studies found that high production cow handlers were able to minimise cow stress and achieve good cow performance by constant attention to the behavioural patterns or performance of each individual cow in the herd. Other studies have been undertaken on the 'ideal' type of person to manage cows in the close confines of the dairy shed (Albright and Fulwider 2007). Interestingly, cows responded best to confident introverts (in other words people with the following set of traits: self-reliant, considerate, patient, but difficult to get on with, forceful, suspicious of change, not easygoing and not talkative). People with these traits were more stable and had an air of confidence, which enabled them to develop positive relationships with their cows that benefited their performance.

The behavioural response of cows to their handlers is best assessed by the flight distance, or how close one can approach an individual animal without it moving away; this can vary from almost zero to 6 m. As expected, the flight distance was larger on dairies where there were more negative interactions such as yelling or hitting. Milk production was also lower on these dairies. As already mentioned, fear of humans can account for 20% of the variation in herd milk yield. Therefore, a change in handler has the potential to substantially alter milk yields. Handler interaction also affects aggressive behaviours of the cows; with less fearful cows being less likely to kick the milker, have lower blood cortisol levels and have higher milk yields.

Cows are able to effectively discriminate between familiar and unfamiliar, as well as positive and negative handlers. A detailed study was made of responses by (untethered) dairy cows to either pleasant or aversive handling with results as follows:

Action of cow	Pleasant handling	Aversive handling
Mean entry time to milking shed (s/cow)	9.9	16.1
Flight distance (m)	0.5	2.5
Dunging in milking shed (frequency/h)	3.0	18.2
Free approach to humans (frequency/min)	10.2	3.0

While the above examples are related to free stall and extensive housing systems, studies have also shown that positive handling and good stockperson attitudes led to an increase in milk yields on dairy farms (Hemsworth *et al.* 2002). These results are applicable to all production systems, including tie stall housing, and further support the importance of stockperson behaviour.

4.6.3   Cowpersonship

With the cows generally located in close proximity to the home, dairying offers more opportunities for women to become closely involved in the day-to-day management than with other farming pursuits. This is important in the village life of South and East Asia, where women have traditionally been the homemakers and family rearers. The cultural and religious bonds limiting their contribution to managing the family budget are being loosened in many SHD communities. Redirecting their mothering instincts from children to livestock is seen by many to provide the basic fundamentals of empathising with, hence providing a better level of care to, the dairy herd. There are also gender differences in cows' responses to handling in that women milkers can increase milk yields and quality. Milkmaids were very common in the days of hand milking and now seem to be making a comeback with machine milking. The politically correct term is then cowpersonship rather than cowmanship.

The term 'cowpersonship' could be defined as developing the skills to get to know the individual behaviour of every animal in one's charge and having the ability to recognise small changes in the behaviour of any animal or all the animals collectively. People with good cowpersonship:

- Are perceptive to the conditions from the animal's point of view, in other words they 'think like a cow'. They can use these skills to detect any changes in the health, comfort and welfare of stock and relate them to ongoing cow performance.
- If they see something wrong, it is immediately put right.
- They organise animal flow through the buildings to balance that with any physical limitations of the building as practically as possible.

The key to cowpersonship is observation and willingness to correct the conditions causing any deviation from a normal behaviour pattern. Some animals cope with stressful situations by changing their behaviour, while others simply change physiological reactions, such as heart and breathing rates. Good cow handlers become aware of such differences between individuals, groups and breeds when handling stock. They can then interact with individual animals that require specific attention.

Insufficient walking space, lack of feeding places and cubicles or resting places are all stressors on a farm, and they induce more social competition and more injuries. Lack of experience of the handler can increase the adverse effect of these factors. Albright and Arave (1997) noted that as well as factors like provision of walking and feeding space reducing social stress in cows, it can also be reduced by improving the handler's husbandry skills. Similarly, it is important to improve these same issues for tethered cattle. As highlighted earlier in this chapter and in Chapter 2, suitable resting places, providing the right resources and space, being aware of social behaviour between neighbouring cows, appropriate exercise and hygienic environments all help to improve the welfare of tethered cows, and all of these factors are in the control of the handler.

As indicated in the sections above, good cowpersonship can lead to 20% higher milk yields over a handler with poor skills. The same holds true with young calves and their positive response to rearers with friendly, as against unfriendly, treatment of their young stock. There are also gender differences in cows' responses to handling, in that women milkers increase milk yields and quality.

Cows are normally quiet and thrive on gentle treatment by handlers. Good handlers allow their cows to develop their own individual personalities as long as no special care or treatment is required and they can 'fit into the system' rather than developing the system to conform to the habits of the cows.

4.7   Practical ways to improve cow flow

This section is specifically written for free moving dairy herds.

4.7.1   Poor movement can be solved with simple observation

The smooth and rapid flow in and out of the milking parlour is highly desirable, but determining the cause of cows' reluctance to enter the parlour may require careful or some astute observation and walking through the system at the cow level. Things that distract cows or can cause them to baulk will slow movement; examples include steep declines, a grate over a drain, a water puddle, change in floor texture, a flapping piece of cloth, clanging metal or a change of lighting along the laneway. A walkthrough of the facility considering issues that can cause baulking can help to solve this. Additionally, milking personnel can influence cow movement as well as the ease of milk harvesting.

4.7.2   Improving cow flow

Well-designed cowsheds and handling facilities can make a difference together with cow management by complementing the natural 'following' behaviour of cattle. Clear entrances and exits allow stock to see and follow others. Good design can also partially compensate for poor stock handling practices by removing the need for handlers to interact with the stock frequently or on an individual basis. We need to use our knowledge on how cows perceive their surroundings to improve cow flow. Based on the sensory abilities and behaviours we've discussed so far, the following considerations will help to improve cow flow:

- Provide wide, clear, well-lit pathways for cow movement.
- Cattle are attracted to the sight of others moving ahead so visual contact needs to be maintained and not obstructed.
- Curved races, with an inner radius of 3 to 4 m, are most useful in situations in which stock are required to wait in queue rather than run feely through the race.
- Races with clear, unobstructed views towards the exit or where animals are meant to move will encourage them to move.
- The sight of stationary cattle adjacent to a race will slow down movement, so it is best to screen race walls adjacent to other animals.
- Keep surfaces as consistent as possible because changes in race construction material or floor type (e.g. slats to concrete) will inhibit cow flow.
- Avoid contrasting colours in yards, raceways and the dairy.
- Ramps with covered sides will not allow stock to judge the elevation and so improve cow flow.
- Provide an incentive for cows to move through the milking parlour, food at the end works particularly well.
- Avoid sudden changes in lighting, floor surfaces and textures, floor level and fence or wall types.
- Avoid changes in critical points along the route, such as at gates, pen exits, corners and entrances to the race or laneways.
- Avoid moving and flapping objects, and noisy and dusty environments. These will all cause animals to baulk.
- Remove any solid projections or obstructions from the cows' path.
- Avoid places where painful procedures have previously occurred.

4.8   Recent behavioural problems arising in cattle

The intensification of cattle housing and management contributes to behavioural problems not seen in grazing animals. Restrictions to normal behaviour via unnatural environmental conditions imposed on cattle by their human caretakers are most frequently at the root of behavioural problems. Cattle, as with other domesticated species, have fewer behavioural problems when left in their natural environment. Therefore, there is a concern that intensive management has resulted in the decline of cows' wellbeing. In some cases, the way that stock behave is the only clue that discomfort and distress are present. This can be all the more subtle with tethered animals.

Restricting natural behaviours to the point of frustration can then lead some cows to engage in apparently pointless behaviour. This can be interpreted as a reflection of reduced activity in intensively managed housing systems. Feeding vices can be attributed to restricting natural foraging behaviour or boredom following a very rapid satisfaction of their nutritional needs. With an understanding of these natural behaviours or instincts that have been thwarted, management can improve conditions for both humans and animals alike. The following is a not exclusive list of common behavioural problems that can be encountered in modern day cattle production systems.

4.8.1 Calves will not suckle

Calves that have gone through the trauma of a difficult birth (dystocia) are more likely than those from a normal birth to refuse to suckle. This delay in suckling is also more pronounced if the mother is a heifer. Since the ability of the calf to absorb antibodies (immunoglobulins) from the colostrum decreases the later it is consumed, and heifers have lower levels of antibodies, any delays in the first suckling are more likely to reduce the quantities of circulating antibodies in the bloodstream of calves. This will reduce the calf's immunity against diseases. This has been discussed in more detail by Moran (2012b). In addition, mis-mothering is more likely to happen when large numbers of cows calve down in intensive dairy systems, which will further add to the problems of delayed suckling and poor immunity status.

4.8.2 Cows refusing to use their stalls

In free stall sheds, cows can refuse to use the stalls if they are not comfortable, are unfamiliar, or are less comfortable than alternative areas. It has been observed that cows rarely use poorly designed and constructed free stalls, often preferring to lie in the dirty walkways. The appropriate dimensions of free stalls are then very important for the size of stock being housed and Albright and Arave (1997) provide a good checklist. In addition, the type of bedding and its thickness can greatly influence stall usage. Some cattle practise 'dog sitting' behaviour in confinement where cows have difficulty in rising or they do this on a regular basis outdoors. This topic is discussed in more detail in Chapter 7 of this manual.

4.8.3 Nymphomania

Nymphomania is linked to a follicular cystic disease of the ovary in cattle. It has a higher incidence in dairy than in beef cattle, probably due to their more intensive housing and management. It appears to have a genetic basis and can be in 5 to 25% of the cows in problem herds. Most cases occur within the first 3 to 8 weeks after calving with the development of the first new follicle. Ovulation fails and in the absence of adequate luteinising hormone, several follicles may grow to form multiple cysts. Cattle so affected may show frequent, intermittent oestrus, stand for mounting and aggressively pursue monosexual 'bulling' behaviour, such as pawing the ground, bellowing and attempting to mount herd mates. Masculinisation of the head and neck, and a prominent tail head are characteristic of the chronically nymphomaniac cow. Manual rupture of the cyst is one of the oldest treatments, although it has risks of haemorrhage and scar tissue formation. Human chorionic gonadotropin and gonadotropin-releasing hormone therapy is used to treat the condition.

4.8.4   Silent heat

This is the failure to indicate signs of oestrus even though the reproductive tract is at the height of influence by the reproductive hormones. Silent heat can be attributed to several factors, including but not limited to: cows being in oestrus but outside the observation period of persons assigned the task of heat detection; movement of cows from pastures to holding yards; slippery concrete and other places of unsure footing; heavy rainfalls; cows with sore feet and lameness; and group dynamics – submissive cows may avoid mounting dominant cows in oestrus. Detection of heat can also be more challenging with tethered animals.

Improving heat detection methods in problem herds is likely to identify cows previously evaluated as being in silent heat. These techniques include combinations of visual observation by trained people, activity meters, teaser bulls fitted with a marker harness, progesterone levels in milk, painting or chalking the tail head, heat mark detectors glued onto the tail head as well as various pressure sensitive transducers attached to radio receivers. Heat can be detected in tethered animals by giving them access to an exercise yard and providing a space where mounting behaviours can be noticed. Pressure testing can also be used for heat detection in tethered animals, where animals that will stand receptively to pressure applied to their back are likely to be on heat.

4.8.5   Aggressive behaviours

As humans are no match for cattle in terms of brute strength, proper respect or caution has to be exercised. Cows are more prone to act aggressively in the first few hours post partum while protecting their newborn from outside intrusion. Cows and heifers on heat or young bulls past puberty may lose their inhibitions towards humans and attempt to mount them.

Dairy bulls have more of a reputation for attacking humans than do beef bulls, this is possibly due to differences in rearing management. Young bulls may initially engage in play behaviour that can escalate into aggressive bunting if the play is not sufficiently discouraged. When entering a bull pen, note possible escape routes that can be taken such as specifically built walk-though gaps in fences. Any bull that has attacked a human should be removed from the herd.

4.8.6 Feed related vices

Feed tossing behaviour is practised by up to 10% of the dairy herd and is exaggerated by the presence of many flies in summer. Cows prefer to eat at ground level where feed tossing is rarely observed rather than from elevated feed bunks. A ritual of rooting, sorting and finally tossing feed along the sides and over the back can lead to 5% feed wastage.

Dropping feed from an elevated feed bunk to the ground may be an animal's solution to fulfilling the natural grazing instinct – that is, putting the feed where it can be more comfortably eaten. The slanted design of headlock stanchions theoretically reduces feed wastage as the animals have to angle their head before leaving, causing the feed to be released back into the feed bunk. Ideally, for new designs, consider lower feeding stations/troughs to accommodate and replicate natural feeding behaviour as best possible.

Water lapping occurs when some cows lick the water with their tongue instead of putting their mouth in contact with the water and syphoning it into their mouth. Excessive water lapping can lead to wet bedding in tie stalls, or formation of muddy bogs around water troughs. The presence of stray voltage may cause this hesitation to drink properly. It might also be a stereotypy with cows in tie stalls, indicating boredom from suppressed grazing behaviour and lack of exercise.

It is important to note that teeth grinding is one sign of pain in cattle and should not be confused with a feeding vice.

4.8.7 Kicking

Cattle can kick backward, forward and to the side with some degree of accuracy and strength. Proper precaution should be exercised, especially with cattle that are infrequently handled. Kicking can be the result of negative temperaments, cattle experiencing fear, or can be an indicator of pain. Identifying which one of these problems is causing the kicking behaviour is important, as cows of poor temperament are not wanted for breeding, whereas the welfare of a cow experiencing fear or pain is compromised.

4.8.8 Changes in normal behaviour

The following would not be described as abnormal behaviour but rather changes in normal behaviour in response to unfavourable stimuli. Cows in unsafe situations exhibit fear, such as those caused by expectations of danger, pain or disaster.

- Increased defecation and urination
- Standing with front feet in stalls and rear feet in walkways
- Increased standing and less lying
- Increased lying time and less frequent standing and repositioning themselves in stalls

- Refusal to use stalls and lying in walkways or partially in stalls
- The 'hesitation waltz' or apprehensive behaviour before actually lying down in stalls. This can take several minutes, in contrast to a few seconds taken by cows at pasture. This intention time is then another measure of stall comfort.
- Unusual actions when rising or trying to rest in stalls
- Lapping at water rather than sucking it up
- Reaching over the walls to drink water rather than stand in the walkway where troughs are located
- Unusual and unexpected approaches to eating or drinking
- Unusual walking actions
- Reluctance to cross gutters or enter some areas of the shed.

This apprehension could be learned from previous experience, originating from a variety of sources of pain, such as:

- Needles or injections given in the milking parlour or at lockups at the feeding face
- Neck rails that are too low, too high or too close to the back of a stall
- Poorly positioned or designed stall partitions

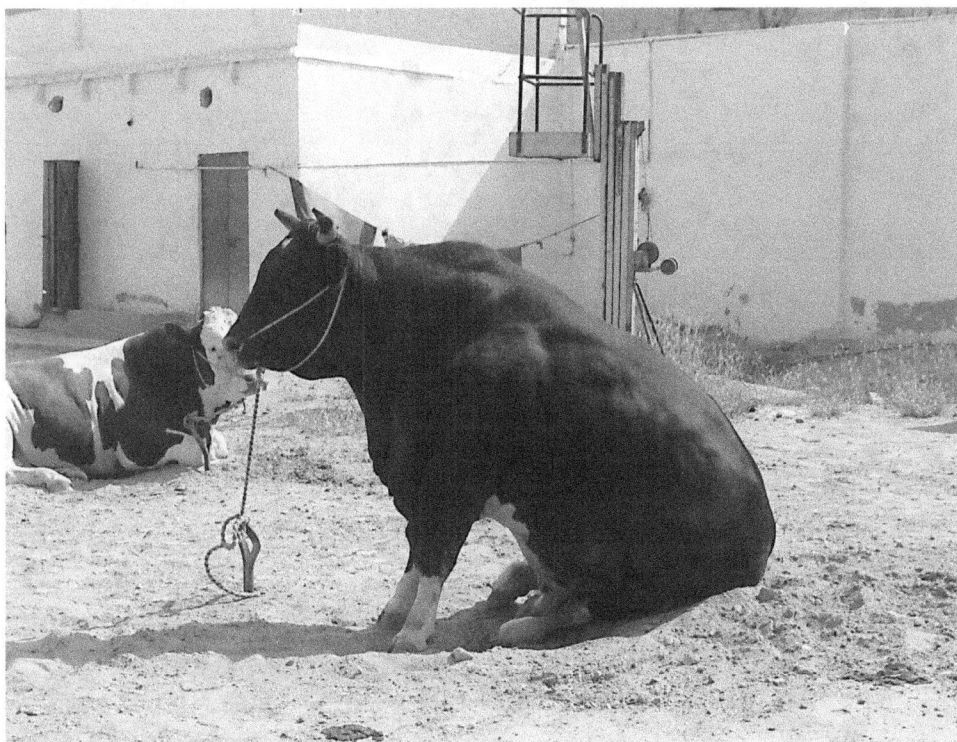

Figure 4.4: A dairy bull 'dog sitting' that could indicate discomfort or pain.

- Hard stall surfaces
- Wide slots in slatted floors
- Flooring surface, either too rough or too smooth
- Obstacles such as walkway manure scrapers, return pulleys on floor scrapers in high traffic areas
- Automatic gates
- Electric crowd gates in pre-milking yards
- Body contact with parts of the milking parlour, especially when stray voltage is present
- Feed bunk barriers
- Electric cow 'trainers', electric wires positioned above stalls to teach cows to step backwards when their back is arched before defecation and urination.

Cows will also show apprehension from cows with dominant behaviour or ones that intrude into their comfort zone. For example, if there are no obvious escape routes or the shed is too dark to make them obvious. Deep gutters and dark alleys and entrances can also 'spook' cows as can frightening objects such as people wearing the same apron or clothes used in milking or while administering painful treatments. Cows adopt avoidance behaviour rather than risk injury.

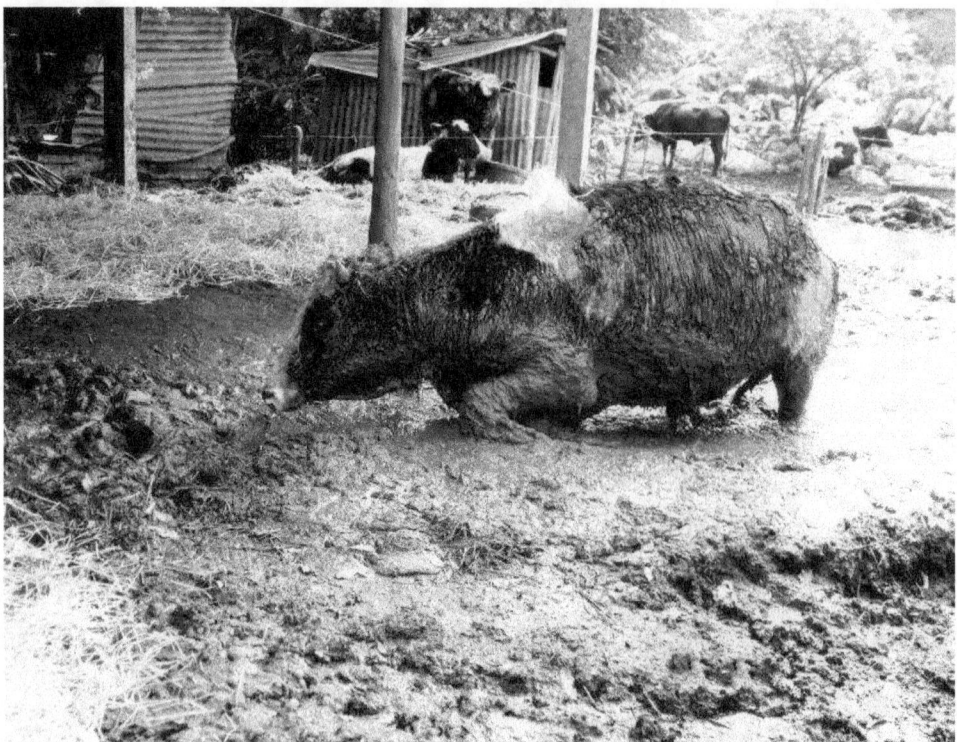

Figure 4.5: This animal is being subjected to very poor stock welfare.

Apprehension may also arise from the design of equipment and facilities that is beyond the ability of the cow to cope with comfortably. Examples are:

- Watering devices that are too difficult to operate, too high or with poor floor access
- Noise from air operating gates and other noisy machinery
- Lack of lighting
- Slippery floor surfaces
- Stall features that contribute to entrapment.

In some free stall sheds, cows lie partially in the stall or completely in the walkway, or they may rise like horses, back into stalls or even paw bedding out of their stalls. In tie stalls, frustrated cows lap at water, chew on water bowls because the stabling and bowl position prevent them from getting their head in to drink comfortably. These cows all show their displeasure with unwanted behaviour. Sometimes, in sheds with slippery floors, they protest silently by not mounting when in oestrus.

In summary, the behaviours of cows will change in response to the situations they are in and the handling they experience, resulting in an increased or decreased frequency of common behaviours (Figures 4.4 and 4.5). Chapters 5 and 6 provide examples of these changes and clarify the situations the cattle are reacting to.

5

Observing cow signals

This chapter discusses the signals that cattle continually give out regarding their health and wellbeing, through their behaviour, posture and physical traits.

The main points of this chapter

- There are three questions to ask when using cow signals to aid farm management decisions, namely, *What do I see?*; *How did this come about?* and *What does it mean?*
- Don't just look, observe and focus these observations by asking: *Is everything as it should be or is there a potential risk in this situation?* Develop an observation routine and use records to aid and interpret any observation and follow-up actions.
- The three main reasons behind any behaviour are – that it satisfies a need; it is a reaction to a stimulus; or it may be due to a physical urge.
- To a large extent farming is about risk management and we can identify two types of risk, known and unknown. Known risks can be controlled by good management but minimising unknown risks requires alertness and good observations. To minimise any damage, farmers need to be able to respond quickly.
- This chapter assesses cow observations in different farm locations: while grazing; in the shed; at the feed barrier and in the milking parlour.
- Astute farmers know the signs of a healthy cow in that she is alert and active, has a glossy and smooth coat, has a good appetite and drinks well and walks and stands without discomfort.

- The early signs of sickness are often subtle, requiring skill and experience to recognise them – such cows may simply 'look different'. Shallow rumens, sweet-smelling breath, high temperatures and evidence of pain or discomfort are clear indicators and sick cows may often withdraw from the group and lie in a stall.
- The cowshed is a system where various factors interact: the layout (feed barriers, calving pen, ventilation); dimensions (width of laneways, roof height); materials (concrete or rubber floors, straw yards); management (hygiene, feeding, stocking density) and the animal, to mention just a few.
- The physical condition of feet and legs (such as bruises and abrasions) and lying behaviour are good indicators of cow stall dimensions and overall comfort. Lameness is a major problem in sheds with poorly constructed laneways and a poorly designed shed layout.
- Cows must have ample space at the feed barrier to minimise aggression and dominance behaviour. Rumen fill, dung consistency, hoof health, feeding behaviour, feed wastage and rumination are all signs of feeding management. Milk yield and composition are good indicators of nutrient intakes.
- The milking parlour provides an ideal place to assess udder and teat health, hocks and feet integrity and coat cleanliness. How a cow behaves tells us a lot about her emotional state and this state influences milk letdown and is also a good indicator of the mechanics of the milking process.
- Much can be learnt about the wellbeing of calves and the state of the calf shed from a competent calf rearer's sight, hearing, smell, taste and touch.
- Even though the dry period is like an annual 8 week holiday for adult cows, their feeding management is very critical during this period.
- It is important to be able to quantify the degree of heat stress endured by milking cows from both the environmental conditions and the animals' reaction.

5.1   Introduction

Cattle continually give out signals about their wellbeing and health. They do this through their behaviour, posture and physical traits. They also do it via their physiological measures such as breathing (respiration) rate, heart rate and concentrations of many metabolites in their blood. Apart from their respiration rate and possibly body temperature, all other physiological measures require expertise and equipment not normally found on dairy farms. With experience, cow behaviour and signals can become important indicators of their performance and welfare.

As Hulsen (2011, 2013) states in his practical manuals on cow signals, the steps in using cow behaviour in farm management decision-making are:

- *What do I see?* This involves careful observations that should be described objectively and precisely.
- *How has this come about?* Why is this happening? What are the causes?
- *What does this mean?* What should I do? What are the practical solutions to any obvious problems?
- In essence, it is look, think, then do.

The major goals of dairy farming include the prevention of diseases and the improvement of cow comfort and wellbeing, resulting in optimal production. Note this does not mean maximise production because economic logic tells us that the returns from any extra production arising from changes in farm management practices must be greater than their costs. This introduces the concept of marginal costs and returns (in contrast to average costs and returns) and this is fully explained in the book *Business management for tropical dairy farmers* (Moran 2009a).

Many years ago, a wise service provider once told the senior author that 'a good calf rearer knows which calves are going to be sick tomorrow or next week'. This statement can be extended to cover all stock on the dairy farm in that 'a good farmer knows which of his dairy stock are likely to be sick tomorrow or next week'. Knowing this, the farmer can take earlier evasive action to save on veterinary bills and improve the cow's comfort. This early intervention can reduce the impact of the health problem through fewer days sick and fewer days until full recovery, if possible, or culling from the herd, if that is the best business and welfare decision. In addition to animal health issues, astute observations can anticipate other potential farm problems such as overstressed stock or changes in the quality of the feeds on offer. So the challenge is to pick up as many signals as possible before the real problems occur. This is the 'take home' message from this chapter. As a wise farmer told Hulsen (2011), 'not knowing something is forgivable, but not seeing something is stupid'. That might be a bit extreme, but it highlights the importance of developing the skills to become an effective observer.

Another reason for looking at cow signals more purposefully is to overcome the danger of 'farm blindness', that is thinking that what you see every day around the farm is normal. One should always ask what is normal on my farm, and is it the same for all farms? It is essential then to make it a point of including specific observations in your daily routine and discussing such matters with your farming colleagues and service providers. It is also worth visiting other farms to note how their specific observations may differ from your farm.

5.2 Don't just look, observe

Astute observers should take into account:

- Not just looking, but looking and observing. You must notice all the signals that stock give out because they can all provide important information on cow wellbeing and comfort.
- Focused observations. You must look for things to evaluate. Ask the question: *Is everything as it should be or might this situation pose a potential risk?*
- Open-minded observations. Look at things as if for the very first time and forget any excuses and preconceived ideas.
- Comparing your current observations with some form of standard that indicates whether additional action needs to be taken – you will then need to develop some standards for your particular situation.
- Observing from large to small, from many to few and from far to near. For example:
  - ➤ Is the herd uniform in size, coat condition, cleanliness, body condition, abdominal fill? If not, why not? Is any non-uniformity important?
  - ➤ How are the animals distributed within the building (particular cubicles, throughout the laneways, on the periphery of the buildings) and if it is non-uniform, why? Is it important?
  - ➤ How many cows are lying down in the cubicles? While resting, is it close to 85%?
  - ➤ How many cows show abnormal posture while walking? Is it sufficient to cause concern about lameness?
  - ➤ After looking at the big picture, zero in on certain areas of the shed or on specific cows worthy of additional observation.
- Ensuring there is an observation routine in which every animal receives some attention, with cows (milking dry and transition) observed three times daily and heifers and bulls twice daily.
- If possible, take into account cause and effect. For example, if there is a physical deformity, what might have caused it, such as swollen feet and access to concrete floors only?
- In addition to your eyes, nose and hands, 'paper information', namely, records, can greatly add to the usefulness of observations. This highlights the value of good record keeping that can be easily accessed to supplement the physical signals emitted by the cow.
- Designing the shed layout for easy observation, such as having gaps in feed barriers and perimeter fences and a centrally located cattle crush for ease of closer individual animal observation if necessary.

- Recording the key observations and any follow-up actions. Writing things down is recommended as it forces you to describe more clearly what you see. It also facilitates information exchange with farm staff and, if necessary, veterinarians or other professionals.

5.2.1 Differences between animals

Assess whether the herd is uniform or if there are marked differences between animals. Pay attention to:

- Animal development: are heifers much smaller than the cows? If so, focus more attention on heifer rearing.
- Body condition: when more than 10% of the cows are too fat or too thin. This indicates a long-term imbalance between feed intake and utilisation. Focus on trough space, availability of feed during the day, hoof health, the way cows select their feed and dietary fibre content.
- Hair colour, coat shine and cleanliness: a glossy coat is a sign of a healthy animal. A dirty coat is always a bad sign, and can identify such things as the need to change the bedding, scouring from illness or poor ration formation.
- Abdominal and rumen fill: these indicate feed intake over the last 24–48 h. Why did the cows eat less? Are we dealing with a risk group (see below)? High yielding cows and those close to calving must reach their optimal feed intake as soon as possible.
- Other signs: are there common abnormalities in the herd? For example, a consistently located lump on many cows' shoulders could indicate improperly constructed or installed feed yoke, or the cows have to reach too far into the feeding place to get their feed. Ulcers from lying indicate a need to improve or change bedding.

5.2.2 Logic of cow signals

There are generally three reasons for specific cow behaviour, namely:

- It satisfies a **need** and the cow wants something, for example she wants to eat her food, wants to lie down or is just plain curious.
- It is a reaction to a **stimulus**, for example she tries to avoid being physically hurt so she moves away from people or dominant cows or even jumps after touching an electric fence.
- It is due to a **physical urge** caused by pain, disease, hormones or she may be due to calve down.

These help answer the question: *Why is the cow behaving in a certain way?* If you do not know whether such behaviour is normal, compare the cow in question with other cows on your own farm and then those on another farm to assess the possible reasons in a completely different situation. Further details on normal and abnormal behaviours are given in Chapter 4 of this book.

As genuine cow signals are repeated, for example kicking off a milk cluster only once may mean a single cow is overreacting, but does she do it at every milking and if so, why? If it is repeated many times, then there must be a common cause such as over milking, the vacuum level is too high, there are teat injuries or even severe fly irritation.

If a cow looks as if she intends to do something, makes an attempt to do it but then stops, there must be a reason why she did not follow through her intention. What were the circumstances or stimulus or stimuli that made her change her mind? Learning to recognise normal behaviour and then the things that might inhibit this provides valuable information about the underlying relations in a herd, housing or health of a cow.

An observation that defies logic can be an extremely valuable cow signal. Hulsen (2011) calls these unclassified notable observations (or UNO, 'you know'). At first glance these findings may appear to be insignificant, but on reflection and further consideration, the observation can become important. If it can be a potentially harmful UNO, it justifies an explanation. For example, if a particular cow drinks water from dirty puddles, she must be thirsty, so providing additional or more accessible fresh drinking water would solve this problem. When evaluating UNOs, use the same three steps listed above, namely:

- Describe exactly what you see.
- Ask yourself, or someone else, what the cause is.
- Determine what influence the signal has on comfort, health and production, and decide whether or not to take action.

5.2.3   Indicator animals and locations

Indicator animals are those that belong to certain groups of stock on the farm that are at greater risk than others. They are often the first to send out signals indicating something is wrong. Observing abnormal behaviour from members of these high-risk groups can provide advance notice of a problem. For example, high yielding milkers will be the first to show up a problem in the formulation of the ration, through unexpected drops in milk yield.

Indicator animals can also be used to monitor the likelihood of a potential problem occurring on the farm, such as a shortage of forage might first become apparent with the changes in milk yields in heifers in the milking herd. Poor handling may first become apparent when previously bolder cows are slower to enter the dairy.

Risk locations on the farm can identify where stock are more likely to be injured, such as a long rough track where small stones can injure hooves, or the calf shed where sudden changes in weather can upset calf wellbeing.

There are times of greater risk for different stock groups on the farm. These can be related to:

- the season, such as the middle of the dry season when soil moisture levels are at their lowest
- a particular date, such as the first extremely hot day in summer
- stock age, such as at weaning time in milk-fed calves
- stage of lactation, such as when the first insemination is usually due.

Additional observations (and actions if necessary) and routine preventative measures can reduce stress during these times to limit any likely problems (Figures 5.1 and 5.2). Responding rapidly to such problems can prevent serious consequences. So it is important to plan ahead to assess whether everything is as it should be and potential problems can be quickly detected and acted upon.

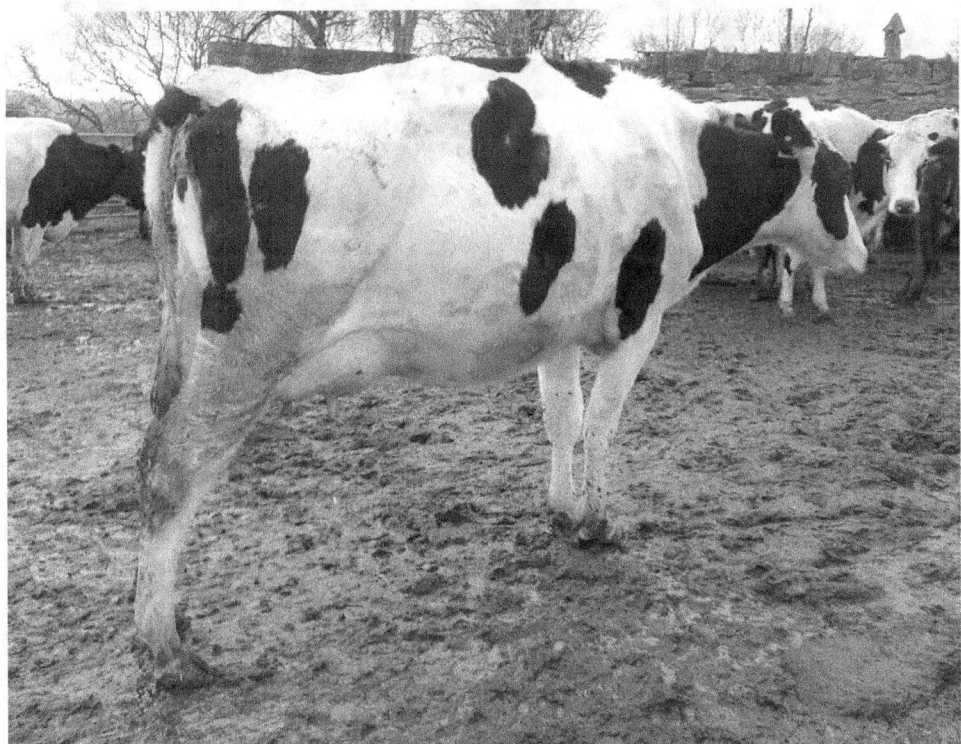

Figure 5.1: Lameness is a major problem on many tropical small holder dairy farms.

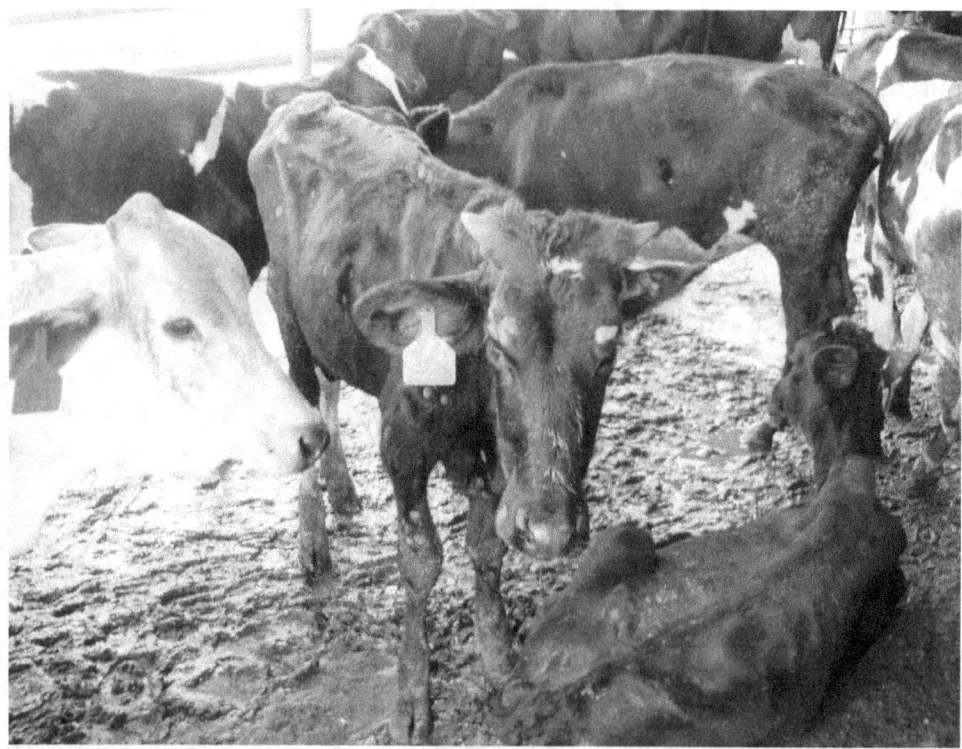

Figure 5.2: These dairy heifers are in appalling body condition and shed conditions.

5.2.4　Risk management

To a large extent, risk can be controlled and we can distinguish two types of risk, known and unknown. Known risks can be controlled by good management strategy. To minimise unknown risks requires alertness and good observations and to minimise any damage, quick response.

Risk management can be broken down to two steps, prevention and damage control. Prevention is reducing the likelihood of a risk occurring, such as:

- Guarantee success, for example, by providing quality forages and feeds.
- Incorporate risk-reducing strategies into daily routines, for example, by calving cows down in a clean, safe and accessible area or maintaining a closed herd by not buying cows in.
- High quality housing and equipment, for example, a well functioning, self-locking feed yoke, or an accessible and well-maintained foot trimming crush with sharp hoof knives at hand.
- Ongoing skill development and effective management, for example, updating technical skills, be willing to change, try and prevent 'farm blindness'.

Damage control is ensuring any damage from the risk is minimised by:

- Identifying the risk through thorough checks
- Acting quickly with strict farm discipline
- Acting effectively through using the necessary knowledge, skills and equipment.

5.2.5 Success factors

Avoiding risks and working out what went wrong are both important steps in improving farm management. But even without doing this, farm management can evolve. A successful farm is not determined by the absence of mistakes but by the proper development of prerequisites for success. Successful entrepreneurs identify and focus on key factors that will lead to success.

These factors depend on the objectives of the business. A high yielding farm with healthy stock and one that produces the bulk of its own forages requires:

- cows with good health, especially feet and legs
- cows with high genetic potential for conformation and production
- cows with capacity to consume and utilise lots of feed
- optimal availability of food with high quality, palatable dietary components in the right proportions
- good housing and outstanding stock care
- minimising heat stress
- high quality risk management.

These success factors need to be routinely monitored to determine whether everything is as it should be (all farm activities, stock health status) and whether this is likely to continue (risk management). The farm can develop into a first rate operation by:

- eliminating management mistakes, that is, remedying shortcomings
- controlling risks and paying closer attention to those areas needing improvement
- concentrating efforts to finetune the success factors in the entire farming business.

Hulsen's (2011) book has many 'take home messages' and the key ones have been summarised as 'one liners' in Box 5.1.

5.3 Cow signals while grazing

Observing grazing stock gives a good insight into their normal behaviour and needs. The way a cow walks; her rumen fill; if she's standing alone – all are signals that could indicate a need to keep a closer eye on individuals or groups of animals.

Box 5.1: 'One Liners' about how cows and humans communicate with each other

- Don't just look ... observe.
- Like cows, use all your senses when observing; ears and nose as well as eyes.
- What do I see, why has this happened, and what does it mean?
- Observe from large to small, from many to few, from far to near – then do this in reverse.
- If cow signals are genuine, they will be repeated.
- Why is a cow doing this? Does it satisfy a need, is it a reaction to a stimulus, is it due to a physical urge?
- Cows are herd animals, so tend to do things simultaneously, but they also form smaller groups within herds, generally based on social order.
- Cows use subtle signals to indicate their social 'class' or ranking (dominance or submissiveness).
- Conflicts often occur between cows of similar rankings.
- Cows tend to moo when they are on heat or are hungry.
- Each cow has a personal space and this varies in size between breeds and their feelings of security and trust.
- Cows feel secure when they know they have plenty of feed, they have escape routes and they know the person handling them.
- Cows feel insecure on slippery floors, when they are very lame and when in the presence of unpredictable personnel.
- The presence of cobwebs in the cowshed is indicative of low air movement, hence poor ventilation.
- If more than 10% of the resting cows are standing, stall comfort needs to be improved.
- When cows lie down, up to 30% more blood circulates through the udder.
- Ration formulations rarely correspond to what cows actually consume – they act only as a starting point and need to be verified and modified on the farm.
- The body language of the cow is the best management adviser – if you can read the cow, you know what to do.
- Cows will tell you what they want.

Although pasture is the most natural environment for cattle, it is still necessary to consider the cow's comfort. Certain aspects are beyond the farmer's control such as excess sun, wind and rain and dampness. For these constraints, cows should be provided with shelter. At the very minimum, they must always have a dry area where they can lie down.

When cows lie down at pasture their behaviour provides a lot of information about their wellbeing. Lame and stiff cows lie in less upright positions and they have a much greater tendency to lie on their side compared to healthy cows. They also hold their head lower.

5.3.1　Leg and hoof health

Pasture provides the best environment for cow hooves as the ground is soft and provides a good grip. But long distances to walk and hard tracks with rough surfaces can still lead to hoof and feet problems. When walking over rough surfaces, hooves are worn down and injuries can occur, especially during wet periods when hooves are softer. The social order, particularly when cows are walking in a line, can disrupt movement when dominant cows push and even bring the line to a standstill. Driving cows in an impatient way leads to fighting and sudden movements and may even frighten cows. If the cows don't have time to see where they are putting their feet, this can cause physical damage. Uneven wear also leads to lameness problems when the outer claw grows faster than the inner claw, resulting in greater weight being placed on the outer claw.

Lameness can be evident when the cow is standing, due to pain in the leg bones and joints. Moving is not painful but bearing weight is and the cow swings the foot forward smoothly but then tries to avoid putting weight on it. Lameness can also only be evident when the cow is moving and this is caused by pain in the tendons or muscles. The animal tries to move the leg as little as possible but does not have difficulty bearing weight. There can be combinations of these two types of lameness.

The degree of lameness can be quantified using a five point lameness/locomotion score, which is described in Chapter 6. Lameness scores in individual cows can be used to select cows for hoof examination before they become clinically lame. Lameness scores for groups of cows or the entire herd are related to cow performance. The higher the lameness score, the greater the reduction in feed intake and milk yield and the poorer the body condition.

5.3.2　Signals of good and poor health

When assessing cow health, proceed from large to small. It is best to observe with an open mind rather than make judgements or excuses. Having someone else come and look with you can help you see more and draw better conclusions.

Signals of good cow heath include:

- The cow is alert and active, she does what she wants to do and is aware of her surroundings. Her eyes and ears are attentive and she is curious about noise and other stimuli.
- She has a glossy, smooth, clean coat without any blemishes. Cows that do not feel well soon lose the shine from their coat and the hairs of their coat may stand on end.
- She has a good appetite and drinks well. Food intake is evident from the rumen and abdominal fill. If food intake is poor for a long time, the cow will lose weight and eventually lose body condition. When she is not drinking enough

or is losing excessive fluids, the eyes become sunken and the skin becomes tight.

- She walks and stands without any signs of pain or discomfort. When in pain or lame, a cow arches her back. Irritation in the pelvic area causes the cow to hold up her tail. If having difficulty walking, the cow first makes movements indicating she is about to walk, followed by obvious head movements when she starts walking.
- The cow is well cared for, with good housing. Cow signals such as overgrown hooves, mange and lice are indicators of poor care and should have been attended to much earlier. Unclipped udders and backs, and dung caked on the cow's skin all suggest a lack of care.

There are eight scoring systems mentioned in this chapter that quantify cow wellbeing and health. These are locomotion/lameness, hooves, legs, cleanliness, rumen fill, dung, body condition and teats. Full details of all these systems are described in the next chapter. Appendix 3 provides a summary of good cow health and welfare while Appendix 4 provides a summary of poor cow health and welfare.

Farmers often notice sick animals because they look slightly different from other stock in the group. The earliest signs are subtle, requiring skill and experience as well as effort to recognise them. It is important to look specifically at animals in risk groups and at risk times.

Cows in negative energy balance have elevated levels of acetone in their blood, milk, urine and on their breath. Some people can smell acetone, even when several metres from the cow.

A high body temperature is an early and clear sign of disease and is part of the immune response and inflammatory process. A cow that is sick but not running a temperature may have a digestive disorder or could be in shock, which occurs when blood circulation is failing. In that case, the cow is cold to the touch especially her ears, lower limbs and udder. Taking her temperature should be the first step in any diagnosis.

When in pain, stock try to reduce the pressure on the sore part, take shallow and rapid breaths and are less aware of their environment. They also eat and drink less, showing signs of dehydration. They will often withdraw from the group and if they are in the shed, they will lie in a stall. Lame cows are more easily startled because they are less able to get away and this becomes very obvious on slippery floors.

5.4   Cow signals in the cowshed

The cowshed is a system where various factors interact: the layout (feed barriers, calving pen, ventilation), dimensions (width of laneways, roof height), materials (concrete or rubber floors, straw yards), management (hygiene, feeding, stocking density) and the animal, to mention just a few. Lame cows place a higher demand on the floor area and the stalls than do healthy cows, and need more space to move. The availability of forages and concentrates influences the social order in the herd and therefore the need for space.

So what standards should a good facility try to achieve? Ultimately, there is one constant factor that determines this standard, namely, the cow. People translate these cow requirements into specifications on the building plan. As cows, their diets and people change, the norm needs to be modified continually. The best solutions are found by weighing up the pros and cons and making a compromise between too much or too little. These decisions are often reached with the aid of specialists, together with good farm sense.

5.4.1 Space and social order

There should not be anything to prevent the cow having easy access to her food, the drinking water or her bed. Every animal needs a certain amount of space in order to feel comfortable. For example, cows need to have enough room to pass each other without touching and they should be able to escape and find a safe haven. Cows with horns increase the need for space and escape routes.

Every herd has a complex social order. There are small groups with bosses and their subordinates and leaders and followers. Bosses are those animals that are allowed to eat first, while leaders initiate activities. A dominant cow forms a serious obstacle to a low ranking animal, which will only pass the more dominant cow if she feels safe to do so. She needs to be able to escape and in order to do that, must have enough space, healthy feet and legs and sufficient grip on the floor. Cows that are lying down do not participate in the competition for social order.

The most common cause of fighting is competition for feed; this occurs when palatable feed is not available throughout the day. In the struggle to get to the tastiest feed, the lower ranked animals will always end up eating second. First-calf heifers have a low social rank and don't know all the cows in the herd. Due to their timidity, they lose out when competing for feed.

Along with visually observing social interactions, things like rumen fill, milk yield, and long bouts of standing, rather than eating or resting, all provide good information about the comfort within the herd.

5.4.2 Shed design and construction

Every shed has its own risks and risk locations. By observing every location in the shed thoroughly, with and without the cows, you can prevent many problems. Risks are found not only in certain areas but also in certain circumstances. These include changes in the weather, hot weather with high humidity, when mixing groups (such as heifers and dry cows), general unrest in the shed, cows on heat, a relief milker, drying cows off and changing ration formulations.

Cows like to drink water without being interrupted so water troughs should not be located too close to feeding areas. If so, low ranking cows would hesitate to drink when thirsty. Locating troughs sufficiently high so cows cannot defecate into the water is not such a good idea because cows like to drink on the level and the steps up to the trough put extra pressure on the hooves.

Cows are sensitive to the amount of light in the shed. They have a reflective layer at the back of their eyes which enables them to see better in dim light. However, they need a lot more light to stimulate their biorhythm than for ordinary sight. Being daytime creatures with a temperate seasonal rhythm, the winter (16 h dark and 8 h of light) is the natural time for them to be dry while the summer (14 to 16 h of light and 6 h of uninterrupted darkness) is optimum for lactation. These conditions stimulate milk production, the animals feel well and are more likely to show signs of heat. Such wide variations in daylength do not occur in the tropics and so diurnal rhythms play little part in their physiological responses to the tropical climate.

Cows perform best within a predetermined temperature range. Below –5°C cows use energy to maintain body temperature while above 20°C they use energy to remain cool, and above 25°C feed intake begins to decrease. When showing signs of severe heat stress, cows with high respiration rates prefer to stand, sometimes with their front end higher than their rear end. This is so the intestines put less pressure on the diaphragm and the cow can breathe more easily. Ventilation is important, particularly around the head, to facilitate air exchange from the lungs. Heat stress is one of the major constraints to small holder dairy (SHD) systems in the tropics with inadequate ventilation restricting heat dissipation in many of the sheds. Roof heights are frequently too low and lack of open sides restricts air movement in sheds. Fans are only occasionally incorporated into ventilation systems while sprinkler systems are rarely installed.

On tropical SHD farms, floors are mainly concrete and all too often they are not roughened or grooved. The majority of effluent disposal is by hand using shovels and scrapers. Despite the fact that there is adequate water in areas with high rainfall, it is rarely used to wash down floors. Consequently floors are often slippery, thus reducing a cow's self-assurance and confidence when moving around the shed. Cattle may well have difficulty performing their natural behaviours such as self-grooming and mounting when a cow joins a sexually active group of cows. Hoof health also suffers as burdens of infection are high and hooves are kept moist on the faeces-contaminated floors. The lack of rubber mats or other soft bedding restricts the use of free stalls for lying down and even in tie stalls cows will not rest for sufficiently long periods.

Slippery floors lead to many signals of discomfort in cows, such as slipping when being rounded up or when taking evasive action and can lead to poor expression of heat. Cows look for less slippery areas in laneways, walking carefully with legs placed apart and heads low and taking small steps and negotiating corners with care. Cows are generally more apprehensive, while low-ranking cows and heifers look for safe havens such as in dead-end laneways.

Obviously the state of the hooves and legs are also prime determinators of how stock cope with floor surfaces in sheds. Scoring systems for hooves and legs are described in the next chapter.

5.4.3 Stalls or cubicles

Cows like to lie down for up to 14 h per day. Lying down is important because the cows can rest, their feet can rest and can dry off and there is more space available for other cows in the laneways. It also increases blood flow through the udder (by up to 30%) thereby increasing the flow on precursors to produce milk.

The lying periods fit in between the periods of feeding and standing. A lying period typically lasts 30 min to 3 h, so the cow stands up and lies down many times each day. During the long lying period in the middle of the day or during the night, she rises, stretches and lies down again immediately, usually on her other side. Cattle spend half their time lying down and they lie down and get up around 16 times every day. When a cow lies down, she puts two-thirds of her weight on her front knees, and they drop freely from a height of 20 to 30 cm. It is therefore very important to have good quality bedding so she can painlessly lie down whenever she wants to. If she takes longer than 5 min on average, you should check the stall and bedding for reasons why she does not lie down immediately.

If stall comfort is not optimum, cows will not lie down unless they are very tired. They are then more likely to lie down for longer than normal and will eat and drink less. In addition, certain problems will soon start to appear – such as swollen hocks. If more than 10% of resting cows are standing, stall comfort needs to be improved.

Stalls are the compromise between space and hygiene. When a cow needs to defecate, she passes dung regardless of where she is. For good hygiene, which will help to prevent udder infections, it is essential that cows do not defecate in stalls and that they are cleaned out several times each day. Small heifers will always defecate in their stalls. Poor stall design can make standing up or lying down difficult. If this is the case, the cows will lie down for abnormally long periods and could have injuries to their knees and hocks. Difficulties when getting up can lead to damaged teats. The stall floor is also important – it should be soft with sufficient grip. Sand or a layer of sawdust (more than 10 cm deep) is the most comfortable.

A brisket locator prevents the cow from lying too far forward in the stall. It should be rounded, with a little give and not too high (say 10 cm). Head rails should not hinder the cow when she stretches her head. Therefore, they should be positioned at less than 20 cm or higher than 90 cm. The dividers should encourage the cow to lie straight, without risk of bruising.

Injuries that indicate that stall design needs improving include:

- **Bruises**: These result from forces at right angles to the hock and occur when the cow lands heavily on the stall floor and from the pressure on the hock when lying down and getting up. The stall surface is too hard or there is insufficient bedding.
- **Abrasions**: These result from forces parallel to the skin over the hock and may indicate that the stall surface is too rough or too slippery, the bedding is too coarse or the stalls were badly built.

Factors that make stall comfort worse:

- **Wet stalls** that soak the skin and lead to hair loss. In addition, skin infections will develop more easily.
- **Acidosis and related problems** cause laminitis due to toxins in the blood damaging small blood vessels particularly in the hooves and joints. This results in pain and a stiff gait and cows have difficulty lying down and standing which leads to bruised hocks.
- **Lameness and leg weaknesses** cause greater difficulty in lying down and standing so cows will have to use their head as a counterbalance even more than normal. Cows are then likely to end up falling forward. They also land heavily and develop abrasions from the stall floor.
- **Large and heavy cows** need a lot of strength and space to stand up and lie down.

Further details of the physical facilities involved in cow comfort are presented in Chapter 7.

5.5   Cow signals at the feed trough

Cow nutrition focuses on achieving maximum dry matter intake and a healthy rumen. There are many factors contributing to rumen health. Nutritionists tend to focus on issues such as ratio of energy to protein and ensuring the ration has sufficient fibre and minerals. However, astute farmers should consider all the factors that can influence a cow's eating behaviour.

Calculated rations rarely correspond exactly to what the cow actually consumes, because of natural variation and the need to make assumptions. Therefore, the ration calculation only acts as a starting point, which needs to be verified and possibly modified in the shed.

When evaluating nutrition, health and production, you need to look to the past as well as the present with the aim of achieving even better results in the future. Information from the past helps you to learn and to understand the current situation. It can be used as the basis for setting new goals such as 'next year I want to produce 50 L more milk per cow and also halve the feet problems'. The cow signals you notice can be used to evaluate the current situation.

Overcrowding at the feed bunk results in increased aggression between cows. This leads to hoof damage and lameness as less dominant cows try to avoid dominant animals by turning away from them, causing them to twist their rear feet on an abrasive surface (concrete). Increased aggressive interactions can lead to even more severe claw damage. The potential for laminitis also increases as cows may consume fewer, but larger, meals or even have reduced feed intakes and spend more time on concrete rather than lying in the stalls. Headlocks reduce this aggression and improve access to feed by socially subordinate cows during peak feeding periods, by offering some physical separation between adjacent cows.

5.5.1 What signals to look for

A high yielding cow giving 30 L/day of milk has a rumen volume of 150 to 200 L and each day, consumes about 22 kg of dry matter and passes about 35 kg dung.

When looking back, important cow signals include:

- changes in body condition scores
- annual and monthly production figures and milk records
- number of metabolic diseases, such as displaced abomasum, milk fever and ketosis
- total number of illnesses
- number of cows culled with the reason for culling
- fertility records.

When assessing the situation and making changes, the important cow signals (and what they indicate) are:

- rumen fill (feed intake and rate of passage)
- milk production today and yesterday (feed intake and energy to protein ratio)
- dung consistency (feed intake and digestion)
- selective feeding (well mixed ration and palatability of ingredients)
- daily feed residues (should be 5 to 10% of feed offered)
- feed wastage (feed intake and selective feeding)
- chewing the cud or rumination (fibre)
- hoof health (locomotion score)
- heat stress.

Close investigation of the cow's body condition around the abdomen can provide a guide as to how much a cow has eaten today, this week and this month (Hulsen 2013).

- A cow that has eaten well has a good rumen fill, belly fill and body condition.
- A cow that has not eaten enough **today** has a reduced rumen fill. This is apparent from the depressed left flank, located at the back of the ribs under the rear lumbar vertebrae, just in front of the cow's hip and is more fully described in Chapter 6.
- A cow that has not eaten well this **week** has a reduced belly fill. This is apparent from the depressed abdomen, located midway down the abdomen under the ribs.
- A cow that has not eaten well this **month** has a reduced body condition score, described more fully in Chapter 6.

Milk production data provide valuable information about individual cows as well as groups. The standard values are affected by the genetic potential of the herd as well as the ration. Table 5.1 presents some examples.

5.5.2 Considerations when preparing the ration

Mature cows eat between 7 and 12 meals per day and each meal lasts about 45 min, giving a total eating time of 6 to 8 h per day. Heifers eat more frequently and consume less at each meal. These should always be sufficient fibre in the rumen to correct acidosis caused by rapidly fermenting feeds. Cows should produce a lot of saliva (from rumination) and the rumen wall should quickly absorb the end products of digestion. To maintain a healthy rumen, cows need to eat sufficient fibre, so ideally they should eat forages and concentrates at about the same time. If the ration does not contain sufficient fibre, cows may actively seek out high fibre feeds such as straw or hay. Low fibre rations increase the risk of a very low rumen pH developing which can lead to toxins killing off some of the bacterial microbes.

Table 5.1.   Examples of herd problems as indicated by milk production and composition data.

Problem	Check point
Severe negative energy balance or ketosis	Difference between milk fat and milk protein %: • > 1.0% indicates negative energy balance • > 1 25% indicates ketosis
Acidosis	Low fat %
High incidence of social conflicts	Heifer production below expectation
Low disease resistance in the herd	Disappointing production from older cows Low milk protein in older cows (< 3.2%) Too many sick cows

For fibre to be effective, the particles should be longer than 0.6 cm, so aim to work with forage 4 cm long.

The rumination time provides valuable information on the ration's fibre content and cows should ruminate for 8 to 10 h per day, making a total of 16 h chewing. High yielding cows produce about 300 L/day of saliva when cud chewing is optimal. At any one time, more than 50% of the cows lying down should be ruminating and this should increase to 90% 2 h after feeding. Cows commence rumination about 45 min after eating and will lie down for about three-quarters of their time spent ruminating. Cud chewing sessions last 30 min or more during which time cows chew each regurgitated cud 50 to 70 times before swallowing it. If chewed less than 50 times, this indicates insufficient fibre.

Cows select their feed on the basis of taste and smell, not nutritional value. This is easy to do with dry mixes and when fed particles are long (> 7 cm). Selective feeding can be assessed by eating behaviour (for example, if cows are burrowing into the feed), variations in dung from cows offered the same ration and of course, by comparing the ration on offer with the residues. Cows often use their tongue to pick out long fibres with the shorter pieces dropping out and later, eaten off the ground. This is characterised by cows burrowing holes and then shaking out the feed.

Cows must be able to approach the feed barrier or trough safely and every animal should have enough space to eat in a relaxed manner. A space for every cow in the herd is an ideal, however, being herd animals, cows all like to eat at the same time. The competition at the feed barrier means that cows will be in a hurry to eat and may not consume enough at any one meal. Separating out first-calf heifers from older cows will reduce this competition and lead to lower risk of acidosis and higher milk production, as they will be more relaxed when eating, thus will eat smaller meals more often.

Unlimited access to drinking water is just as important as providing sufficient fresh feed. Cows like to drink fast, up to 20 L/minute. If they cannot, their water intake will decline and their feed intake and milk production will suffer. Every 1 kg feed dry matter utilises 5 L water and a 40% decrease in water intake can cut milk yield by 25%.

Cows prefer to drink from a large water trough at a low level and like to be able to stand quietly and safely while drinking. They will always choose the freshest and cleanest water. Cows commonly drink when they get up from resting, after eating and again after milking. Water troughs should then be placed in many positions throughout the shed and close to the feed barriers. As a rule of thumb, one large trough should be provided for every 20 cows or one smaller one per 10 cows.

5.5.3   Risk groups

On every farm there are groups of animals that are susceptible to shortcomings in the ration. These groups then require closer monitoring than others. They can also be used as a means of monitoring risks, as indicator animals. Separating risk groups from the rest of the herd reduces the risks. For example, freshly calved cows and heifers should be separated from the rest of the milking herd.

The four main groups of risk animals are:

- **Heifers:** Risks include inadequate feed intake, acidosis and hoof problems. The connective tissue in heifers becomes weak at the time of calving. Rations too high in energy or protein result in udder oedema and soft hooves. If the mineral ratio is wrong, this may also contribute to oedema. In addition, these animals may not eat enough forage compared to concentrate, a particular problem with insufficient space at the feed barrier. This can lead to laminitis. The combination of weakened connective tissue and laminitis increases the probability of hoof problems.
- **Freshly calved cows:** Risks include milk fever, ketosis and fatty liver, metritis and mastitis. If these cows do not eat enough soon after calving, they need extra care and attention. Calving down in a dirty pen can lead to udder and uterine infections.
- **Cows in first two months of lactation:** Risks include inadequate energy intake, acidosis and displaced abomasum. During the first 6 to 8 weeks of lactation, low forage intake can lead to acidosis. The acidic rumen is poorly filled, does not contract and the contents are mushy. The dung shows the signs of poor feed digestion, smells acidic and alternates between thick and thin. Cows do not ruminate properly or for long enough, so often discarded cud is seen in the pen.
- **Cows at end of lactation:** Risks include getting over fat and reducing concentrate intakes too quickly. Condition score, milk fat and protein levels should be monitored. Getting too fat is due to too much energy and not enough dietary protein or a ration that is too rich for the level of milk production.

5.6 Cow signals in the milking parlour

The cows enter the milking parlour one by one and stand for at least 5 min during which time you get a good look at their udders, bellies and legs. Before you put the milk cluster on, you feel the udder and teats and assess the foremilk (strippings). Then you can record how much milk she gave. As a daily routine, milking then provides many opportunities to watch out for cow signals. The better you see the cows, the more information you can gather. If it is difficult to see the cows clearly in the parlour, then you will need to do more monitoring in other places.

For many farmers, milking is the best part of the day as they enjoy the peace and quiet as well as the close contact with their cows. Peace and quiet are good signs in the milking parlour because the cows are also relaxed and it's easier to notice whether they are healthy or showing signs of illness. Restlessness occurs when there is fear or pain or irritation.

Milkers who are relaxed and 'animal focused' enhance the calmness of the cows. Often they have a good feel for the cows and know almost everything about every animal. However, not all farmers have this skill and have to work hard to remember the information. If several people milk the cows, the important information has to be recorded, such as which cows are currently being treated with antibiotics. Hanging a clipboard where it is clearly visible is a simple effective method. It takes time to teach yourself to become aware of things to observe in the milking parlour and you need to develop a good routine. For example, always check the foremilk (strippings), rumen fill, hocks and hooves.

A relaxed milker positively affects the milking process. This has been covered in detail in Chapter 4. The parlour should provide good lighting, particularly at the bottom of the udder, be warm in winter and cool in summer, and be free from draughts to provide a pleasant working environment. A fan provides fresh air, discourages flies and helps to keep any fumes from the footbath out of the parlour.

5.6.1 Cow behaviour during milking

The cows should not be nervous at milking time. Pay close attention to their behaviour, such as how keen are they to come in? If they are nervous, what is the cause? Is milking painful? Do they have unpleasant experiences in the milking parlour? Is the floor slippery? Cows often enter the parlour in the same order, this reflects their social order in the herd. So if a cow does not enter in her normal position, something unusual is probably going on.

Rough handling while rounding the cows up leads to conflict and some cows having to move abruptly. The cows can injure themselves and have hoof problems. They will also become more anxious. Restlessness, fear and pain increase levels of adrenalin and other stress hormones in the blood which will inhibit the release of oxytocin, the hormone that makes cows let down their milk. As well as causing milk letdown and uterine contractions, oxytocin creates a thirst which explains why cows like to drink during and after milking and also at calving.

Cows are creatures of habit so will milk out better if a simple routine is followed when preparing the udder and putting on the cluster, rather than working in a haphazard way. The cow should stand still so that the cluster can be attached quickly without any air being sucked in. The cluster should be attached between 60 and 90 s after pre-treatment of the udder, then the milk should start flowing almost immediately and keep on flowing. Putting on the cluster, milking itself and cluster removal should all take place quietly. If the milker is calm, the cow barely notices the milking process.

If the cow is unsettled and jumpy, there could be a variety of causes, such as pain, fear and demanding concentrates. It could also be due to malfunctioning of the milking machines, the milker being rough, not enough space for the cows to stand, teat injuries, fly irritation or stray voltage on the cluster or other equipment. Defecating and urinating during milking are signs of anxiety. Another signal is how the cow responds to the sucking noise of the cluster. She should not jump. A fearful response might be due to being previously punished for kicking off the cluster.

While she is being milked, the cow will often seem to be in a daze while she may also chew her cud. Feeding concentrates can encourage cows to come into the parlour and will stimulate milk letdown. Be consistent and precise when providing concentrates because cows learn to demand more by behaving restlessly and kicking off their cluster. This behaviour develops because the cow is rewarded with extra concentrate. Some clever cows are even able to operate the concentrate lever themselves.

The rear quarters contain the most milk and at the end of the milking process, all quarters should be milked out. Take off the clusters when the rear quarters are empty; this does not mean that the front quarters have been over milked.

Cows should be able to leave the milking parlour quietly and in a relaxed manner. Jumpy cows and sudden movements are the first signs that they are unsettled. Cows should not have to worry about slipping or being chased when entering or exiting the milking parlour. Sharp bends and slippery floors are risk locations for the cows and make them nervous. Cows also dislike steps, so a slope is a better option, with the milking area at the highest point. Sharp protrusions, electric wires and a traffic jam at the exit all act as obstacles. So avoid risks and remove obstacles.

5.6.2 Cleanliness, hygiene and cow health

Cows have to be clean because good hygiene prevents disease. Dirt is also a negative signal indicating the cow has been or is ill (diarrhoea) or that something untoward has recently happened, such as she fell or was jumped on. If the cows are always dirty, then it is difficult to spot any changes in the degree of cleanliness.

Dirty **udders** and **teats** increase the likelihood of mastitis, which is caused by two types of bacteria. These are first, the contagious bacteria that live on the cow's skin and are transferred from cow to cow in the parlour. The other bacteria are environmental bacteria that live in the shed, stalls and straw yards contaminating the udder there. Dirty udders are hard to clean properly and they contaminate milk with dirt and bacteria. Clipping the hairs off the udder improves the hygiene, ease of working and access to the teats for cleaning.

Dirty hooves indicate either there is a lot of dung on the floors or that it is very loose hence the hooves are wet for a large part of the day. Dirty wet hooves are more susceptible to disease (soft hooves and skin, pathogens in the faeces), will make the footbath ineffective and can be transferred to the teats. Ideally dirty hooves should not be hosed in the milking parlour as this will distribute dirt and manure further in the area via the fine water droplets.

In many milking parlours, the **hocks** are at eye level during milking, making it easy to monitor their health by assessing the number and type of hock injuries. The normal healthy hock is free from skin lesions and swelling. Ideally, the hair coat in that area is smooth and continuous with the rest of the leg. Bald patches are acceptable but bruising and infections cause pain and discomfort, therefore, they are serious signals. The cause is likely to be the stall floors, stall design and/or lameness. In deep sand stalls that are well maintained, it is rare to find any hock showing bald areas or swelling. This, as well as comfort to the cow as seen by lying behaviour, are two of the reasons why deep sand stalls are the most production and welfare friendly bedding.

The bony part of the hock can also become swollen through severe bruising when a fluid-filled cushion forms. This is a sign that the stalls are uncomfortable. Traumatic abrasions from dirty, wet stall floors can cause the skin to become infected and this can extend subcutaneously (under the skin). In severe cases, the joint also becomes infected and very swollen and makes the cow permanently very lame. She must then be culled. Hulsen (2011) sets the herd targets for stall injuries to the hock at 30% for bald patches, 10% for bruises and 10% for skin infections.

What applies to hocks also applies to **hooves**. The top side of hooves can be easily examined in the milking parlour, although the underside is more easily examined in the shed. First assess the overall health, hygiene and cow stance. Look for any signs of pain, swelling around the coronary band (at the top of the hoof tissue) and laminitis. Cows with sore hooves regularly lift their legs and spraying cold water on a hoof with an open wound, often digital dermatitis, causes an immediate pain reaction. For this reason, affected cows will try to avoid footbaths.

Hoof conformation should also be assessed because abnormalities occur through irregular growth or uneven wear. This can be affected by foul-in-the-foot (see Chapter 6), laminitis and genetics. Poor foot trimming can also be the reason for many cows not standing properly. With laminitis, the attachment of the hoof wall to the underlying bone weakens and the hoof tip turns upwards. This is visible as a cleft at the front of the hoof and divergent growth lines up the hoof.

Hoof problems can be minimised by ensuring:

- Low infection rates: keep the floors and hooves clean and dry, treat infections promptly and use preventive footbaths. Also try and maintain a closed herd so as not to import potential hoof problems.
- Good feeding strategy: provide sufficient fibre in the diet to prevent laminitis and ensure the rapidly and slowly degradable ration components are eaten simultaneously.

- Optimum immunity: ensure optimal feeding management, particularly of the transition cows and the integration of first-calving heifers into the milking herd.
- Avoid injury: provide level floors with sufficient grip, with some give (so not too hard) and no loose stones. Ensure good routine foot trimming and aim for peace and quietness in the cowshed.

Ongoing problems with soft, wet hooves require closer attention to make the surroundings cleaner and drier. Aggressive hoof infections require focusing on the sources of infection and on optimum hoof and cow immunity. If there are problems with excessively dry hooves, the best approach is to ensure even load distribution and optimal hoof shape (by trimming). It is generally not advisable to make the surroundings damper because this can increase the infection pressure. Hoof disorders can occur due to constant exposure to adverse conditions such as a continuously wet floor, but short-term factors can also be a cause, such as a heavily contaminated area of the shed. Faecal material and moisture are risk locations for hoof infections.

Rumen fill can also be assessed during milking as it provides a good opportunity to assess the volume of the rumen contents, which is a guide to the content and thickness of the fibre layer. Cows standing with their left side towards the handler will provide an excellent view of the rumen, but with practice, a view of the right side will also prove useful. Depending on the length of milking, the last cows' rumens will not be as full as the first cows'. Stage of lactation is also going to vary the rumen fill. Maximum dry matter intake should be reached by 10 weeks post-calving. The rumen scoring system is fully described in Chapter 6.

Milk quality: It is important to routinely evaluate the integrity of the milk before putting on the milk cluster. To closely examine milk, first extract some by hand milking as foremilk, discard the first few strips as they just flush away the bacteria in and around the teat opening. If there is something wrong with the milk, small clots of milk protein are easily seen. In severe cases, these may also contain blood proteins that have leaked into the milk through blood vessel walls in the mammary tissue. Mastitic milk (even subclinical) has a higher salt content than normal milk, hence it has a higher electrical conductivity when tested. If clinical mastitis occurs due to late diagnosis, other cows are more likely to become infected. Blood clots and red colouration caused by burst blood vessels are more common in heifers because the udder is still growing rapidly and there is udder oedema. Sometimes the symptoms occur through the cow slipping and falling over. This bleeding generally stops on its own accord.

For the **teats**, milking is an intensive process. Healthy teats and a well-functioning machine are the prerequisites for success together with correct teat shape, proper teat placement and appropriate milking speed. The teat end together with the teat canal form a crucial barrier against invading bacteria. Forces on the teat end during milking cause calluses to develop and if the skin around these calluses becomes roughened rather than remains smooth, udder infections and mastitis are more likely to occur. Such infections can be caused by:

- vacuum level being too high
- pulsation rate is not properly adjusted
- cows are milking for too long
- continued milking when the quarter is empty (over milking)
- rubber liners don't fit, due to abnormal teat shape or wrong liners
- rubber in the liners is damaged and the liners feel roughened due to delay in replacing them.

After milking, good teats are flexible and naturally coloured. The teats should be dry when the cluster is removed. If they are wet, the milk is not being removed quickly enough from the cluster and it is shooting back and into the teat. This creates the risk of the udder becoming infected with bacteria from the teat skin or from a previous cow.

If the liner fits properly, the vacuum is much lower at the top of the cup than at the teat end. With small teats, such as in heifers, and liners that are too large or wet from preparing the cow for milking, the vacuum can be excessive at the teat end. This can cause small haemorrhages in the skin and the cows become unsettled due to painful teat ends.

The 'pinch line' where the rubber liners come up to on the teat, is the result of the teat being stuck on the liner. This is caused by a liner that is worn out, stiff or too wide, or a pulsator that has an excessive rest phase. The teat score provides some degree of objectivity when describing teat health and is described in Chapter 6.

5.7 Signals given out by calves and heifers

Dry cows and heifers are high risk animals as they go through many risk times and may not receive enough care when the farmer is busy. This is unwise given that future herd performance depends on these cows. Times of risk include birth, the first few days of life, disease outbreak in calves, moving, weaning, ration changes, mixing groups, certain types of weather and climatic changes, a different handler and transportation. Other more farm-specific risks become apparent on closer inspection and when planning future management strategies.

The first few days of life are a challenging time for all newborn calves. They must get sufficient colostrum (5 L on the first day with at least half of this during the first 12 hours). This, together with clean, comfortable housing, are the keys to success during the first month of life. The best signals of quality calf care are:

- number of cases of diarrhoea
- mortality rate (also record the age)
- number of navel infections
- growth and feed intake.

The senior author has written a book specifically on young stock management on tropical dairy farms (Moran 2012b). This book contains considerable

Table 5.2. Using your senses to monitor the wellbeing of calves and conditions in the calf shed.

Senses	Indicators of wellbeing
Eyesight	Bright and alert eyes Droopy or upright ears Soft and shiny skin and coat Panting and rapid respiration rates Abnormal discharges from eyes, mouth or body Whether navels and joints are swollen State of faeces residues on calves' back legs (colour and consistency) State of faeces on floor (runny, too clumpy) Any excess feed residues Willingness of calves to eat and drink Any abnormal calf behaviour Proportion of calves resting, standing or moving around If calves stretch when they get up General state of calf shed (drainage, ventilation) General tidiness and cleanliness of calf shed
Hearing	Grinding of teeth Bellowing Laboured breathing Coughing Unsettled calves moving around pens Dripping taps or water troughs
Smell	Abnormal odour of calf's breath Odour of faeces Any other abnormal calf odours (infected hooves) Odour of whole milk or CMR powder Odour of bedding Odour from mouldy feeds Odour of air, hence state of ventilation Odour coming from poor drainage
Taste	Taste of whole milk or calf milk replacer solution Taste of concentrates and forages
Touch	Whether noses are dry Whether ears are warm, hot or cold General level of heat or cold stress for calves Any abnormal draughts Whether air is too damp, indicating poor ventilation Temperature of milk or calf milk replacer solution

information about many aspects of calf and heifer rearing, with one chapter (Chapter 12) specifically on calf and heifer signals called 'Communicating with the calf'. It contains Table 5.2, which provides some insight into how humans can use their six senses to assess how well the calves are coping with their shed environment.

5.8 Signals given out by dry cows

For the milking cow, the dry period is like an 8 week annual holiday. The first few days are stressful because of the changes in management, specifically the previous twice daily milking. This is followed by a period of rest and contentment. But at the end of this dry period, the cow must be completely ready for the recommencement of her duties in the milking herd but in addition, she must give birth to her calf and then immediately return to milk production. The cow's body condition should hardly change during the dry period yet she must eat sufficiently to maintain it. Ideally there should be daily evaluations of rumen fill, feed residues and dung and weekly assessments of body condition.

The period around calving time represents the time of greatest risk in the cow's life. Adequate preparation and outstanding care are key factors if this transition period is to take place with minimum problems. Usually the cow will pass through two groups during their dry period. First, she will be classed as a 'far-off cow', from drying off to 3 weeks before calving. Then she will become a 'close-up cow' for these last 3 weeks. This is part of the transition period, from 3 weeks before until 3 weeks after calving.

5.8.1 Transition period

Targets at the beginning are:

- body condition score of 3.5 points out of 5, or 5 points out of 8
- maximum feed intake; check rumen fill and weigh feed
- proper mineral balance; undertake blood and urine analyses
- healthy feet and legs; use leg, hoof and locomotion scores
- good overall health; cow is alert.

During the transition period, aim for:

- optimum ration; check ration formulation, dung score, disease status
- continuous availability of palatable feed and water; check rumen fill, water troughs, feed intake
- outstanding hygiene; check cleanliness scores and shed
- comfortable stalls, spacious and well-ventilated housing; check lying behaviour, space and climate control

- minimal stress; check gradual changes in management and also behaviour
- good quality care and control of conditions; evaluate care and risk management.

5.8.2 Far-off group

Dry the cow off in one go and hygienically insert a tube of 'dry cow' antibiotic cream as part of the mastitis prevention program. Move her to the resting group where she will be fed a very basic ration but with plenty of drinking water. The feed intake will slowly decrease because the growing foetus is occupying more space in the abdomen.

During the dry period, the teat canal is closed by a keratin plug, which develops over several weeks. However, in about 10% of the cows, the closure is incomplete, bringing a continuous risk of mastitis during the dry period, particularly immediately after drying off and just before calving.

5.8.3 Close-up group

It takes 4 to 6 weeks for the rumen to completely adjust to a new ration, hence the milking cow ration should commence 3 weeks before calving. During the transition period, all types of unrest, discomfort and stress, such as radical changes in housing and feeding and large changes in groupings, are undesirable. Introducing new cows to the close-up group will invariably lead to some conflicts, but after one or two days a new order will be established and peace and quiet will return. Avoid group changes on the day of calving, unless the cow has been isolated to remove any competition.

Just before calving, the udder fills, often with oedema present. The vulva swells and loosens and once the ligaments (running from the spine to the pins beside the tail) are completely slack, the cow usually calves within 24 h. The body temperature also falls by between 0.5 and 1.0°C.

5.8.4 Calving

Check every animal thoroughly at least three times each day and if necessary, intervene quickly and effectively. On the day of calving, use established routines, setting goals and checking whether they have been achieved. If they have not, then improve appropriate management. Such goals include:

- 95% of cows calve in the calving pen
- < 5% have retained placenta at 8 h or more post calving
- < 10% develop metritis
- < 5% develop hypocalcaemia (milk fever)
- < 5% calf mortality within the first 24 h
- < 5% have displaced abomasum.

5.8.5   Post calving

On the day she calves, the cow does not eat much because of the calving process and the associated stress, which is due to social conflicts, deficiencies in the housing and dietary changes. Severe stress can lead to several days of underfeeding. The feed intake on the day of calving is a good indicator of the quality of the dry cow management. The more she eats, the better start she will get to her lactation.

5.9   Cow signals of heat stress

5.9.1   Symptoms of heat stress

There are many symptoms of heat stress, with ones more relevant to shedded cows shown in italics below (Moran 2005). The initial signs are behavioural while the last five signs are the more severe physiological ones due to a failure to cope and therefore requiring immediate attention to reduce their adverse effects on cow performance. In order of increasing severity, they are:

- body aligned with direction of solar radiation
- seeking shade
- *refusal to lie down*
- *reduced feed intake and/or eating smaller amounts more often*
- crowding over water trough
- body splashing
- *agitation and restlessness*
- *reduced or halted rumination*
- grouping to seek shade from other animals
- *open mouthed and laboured breathing*
- *excessive salivation*
- *inability to move*
- *collapse, convulsion, coma*

- *physiological failure and death.*

As well as behavioural symptoms, heat stressed cows will produce milk containing less milk protein or solids not fat. In addition, milk fat levels may decrease if cows markedly reduce their forage intakes.

The severity of heat stress depends on many factors. These include:

- actual temperature and humidity
- length of the heat stress period
- degree of night cooling that occurs
- ventilation and air flow

- cow breed and size
- level of milk production and dry matter intake before heat stress
- housing type, overcrowding, aspect
- water availability
- coat colour, if exposed to sun
- hair coat depth.

Milking cows are maintained in a variety of environmental conditions. Without access to shade, the heat load on cattle grazing at pasture is generally lower than for cattle in dirt yards, because the dirt surface absorbs less heat then grass, thus radiate more heat onto the stock. For example, the surface of a dirt yard can reach 60 to 80°C (on a day with high solar radiation and ambient temperatures of 40 to 45°C), but it will cool down rapidly once the sun sets. Clearly, access to shade, whether at pasture or in yards is highly desirable in regions with high radiation heat loads.

5.9.2 Temperature Humidity Index

The best single descriptor of heat stress is the Temperature Humidity Index (THI), as this combines temperature and relative humidity into a single comfort index. The relationship between temperature, humidity and THI is presented graphically in Figure 5.3 and also in Appendix 1. The higher the index, the greater the discomfort, and from Figure 5.3, this occurs at lower temperatures for higher humidities. Its effect on cow performance is summarised in Table 5.3.

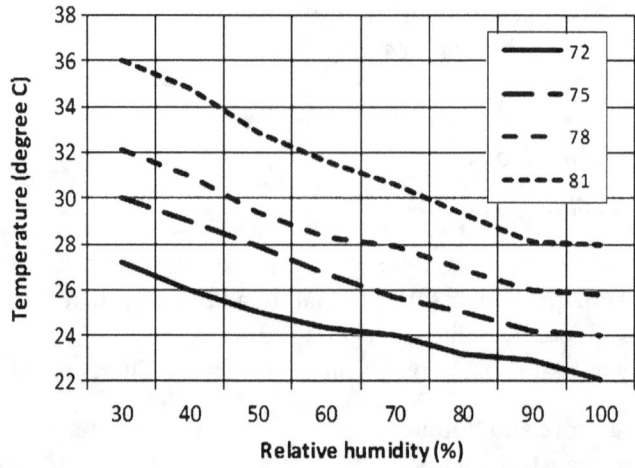

Figure 5.3: The effect of increasing relative humidity on the temperature to produce the same Temperature Humidity Index (72, 75, 78 or 81).

Table 5.3. Effects of Temperature Humidity Index (THI) on dairy cow performance.

Comfort zone	THI	Stress	Comments
A	< 72	None	–
B	72–78	Mild	Dairy cows adjust by seeking shade, increasing respiration rate and dilution of blood vessels. Cow performance is adversely affected with reproduction more so than milk yield.
C	78–89	Severe	Both saliva production and respiration rates increase. Feed intakes decrease while water intakes increase. Milk production and reproduction are both reduced.
D	89–98	Very severe	Cows will become uncomfortable due to panting, high saliva drooling and high body temperatures. Milk production and reproduction will markedly decrease.
E	> 98	Danger	Potential cow deaths can occur.

Comfort zone. A: No stress; B, Mild stress; C, Severe stress; D, Very severe stress; E, dead cows.

Heat Load Index

Meat and Livestock Australia (2006) has developed a Heat Load Index to assess environmental heat load on feedlot cattle. This is based on a combination of measures of heat load, namely:

- black globe thermometer, a measure of radiation heat load which takes into account both ambient temperature and solar radiation
- relative humidity
- wind speed.

The index includes several adjustment factors such as genotype, coat colour, access to shade, water temperature in drinking troughs and whether the animal is sick or healthy. Use of this index over time allows for the calculation of an accumulated heat load and the required heat loss during the night to maintain zero heat balance. However, developing such a Heat Load Index for Asian SHD cows, normally maintained in sheds, is unlikely to provide an additional useful management tool.

Adverse effects of heat stress

For Friesians producing 20 kg/d, a THI above 78 leads to a decline in milk yield. A THI of 78 occurs at 29°C with 50% humidity or at 27°C with 80% humidity. There is also a decline in milk composition (milk fat and milk protein contents) but this occurs at 1–2°C higher than corresponding break points for milk yield.

With regard to reproduction, this declines before milk yield, namely, at THI of 72, equivalent to 25°C plus 50% humidity or 23°C plus 80% humidity. Cows in early pregnancy (up to 3 weeks) can abort while cows in mid-pregnancy can have reduced birth weights. Cows are also more likely to have shortened and/or silent heats (less than 8 h). Heat stress delays heat (hence submission rates) and, at the time of insemination or during the following 3 to 5 weeks, it can reduce conception rates and increase embryo mortality. By comparing conception rates between seasons (hot v cool or wet v dry), heat stress may be diagnosed as a problem if seasonal conception rates differ by more than 10–12%.

Cows are particularly vulnerable at temperatures above 30°C or, above 25°C with high humidity. Cows producing more than 15 kg/d of milk are more susceptible to heat stress due to their higher metabolic heat load. Zebu cows are less susceptible than Friesians because of their dense flat coat and higher density of sweat glands, however, exactly how less susceptible has not been documented. When planning strategies to minimise heat stress, it is then important to give priority to non-pregnant cows, usually in early lactation.

Adverse effects of heat stress are delayed by several days. The effect of mean THI two days earlier has the greatest influence on milk yield, while the effect of mean temperature two days earlier has the greatest influence on feed intake.

Another good 'rule of thumb' when assessing heat stress for dairy cattle is that air temperature (in °C) added to humidity (in %) should be below 90.

Improvements in milk yields of up to 3 to 5 kg/d are possible through effective cooling strategies.

5.9.3   Using respiration rates as a guide to heat stress

Clinical signs of heat stress

The following signs can be used to assess the degree of heat stress:

- Mild heat stress: Drooling, increased respiration to 70–100 breaths/min.
- Moderate heat stress: Drooling, respiration of 100–120 breaths/min and occasional open mouth panting.
- Severe heat stress: Drooling, respiration rate greater than 120 breaths/min and open mouth panting with tongue out. Cattle also have an agitated appearance, hunched stance and will often have their head down.
- Cattle can move from mild to severe heat stress very quickly, within 30 min to a few hours. Therefore extra vigilance is required once mild heat stress is detected.

Monitoring respiration rates

Observing the behaviour of cows is important in deciding when to modify management. If respiration rates reach 70 breaths/min, milk yield and reproduction may be compromised; this corresponds to 39°C body temperature, in

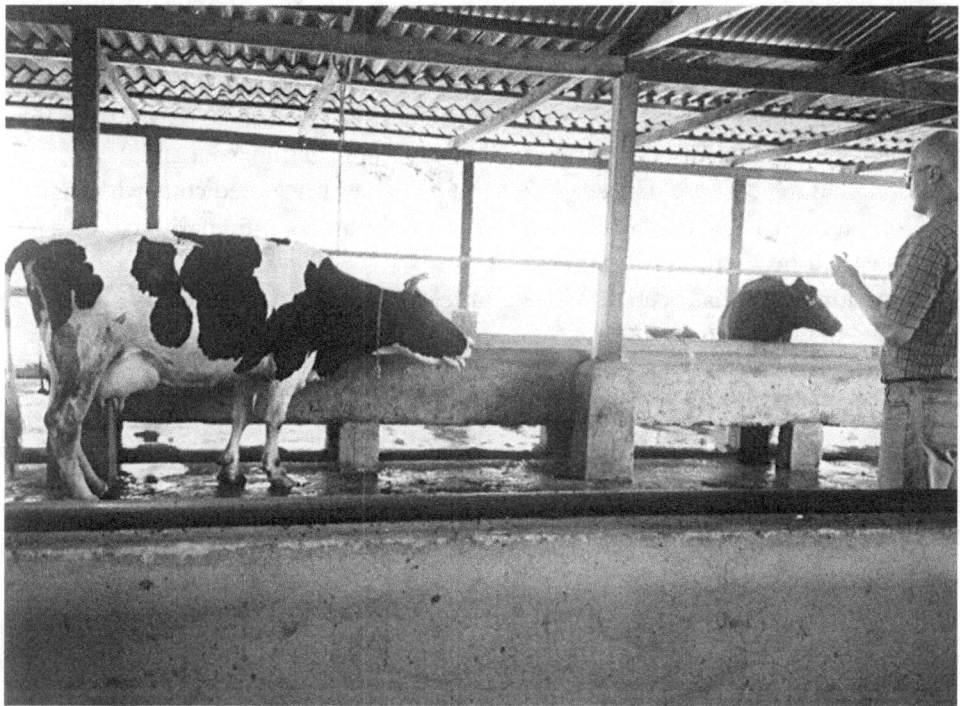

Figure 5.4: Counting respiration rates in a heat stressed cow.

contrast to a normal body temperature of 38.5°C. Higher yielding cows have faster respiration rates, because of the extra body heat production associated with higher feed intakes and milk yields. For such animals, if respiration rates exceed 80 breaths/min in 70% of the cows, it is indicative of heat stress. Certainly, when they exceed 100 breaths/min, cooling strategies should be introduced.

Respiration rates are easy for farmers to monitor. Ensure the cow is standing or lying in a relaxed state and preferably cannot see the farmer (see Figure 5.4). To improve accuracy, the farmer could move his hands in time with abdominal movements until they are at a steady rate. Using a watch, he should count the abdominal movements for 10 s, repeating the exercise to ensure the count is consistent. Multiplying this by six will give the respiration rate in breaths per minute.

Monitoring respiration rates at various times of the day is a useful tool in assessing the suitability of sheds for milking cows. If rates exceed say, 60 breaths/min in the morning, before the shed heats up, it is likely that the cows would benefit from simple modifications in their environmental management. It is unlikely that major modifications in shed design could be justified, such as increasing roof height or pitch or shed height at the side, although serious consideration should be given to constructing roof vents. If minor improvements cannot be made in the shed's natural ventilation, such as removing obstructions to the prevailing breeze, fans and/or sprinklers should be installed.

One enterprising farmer in Vietnam constructed a small shelter away from the cowshed, which maximised natural ventilation through a high roof and its location, making best use of prevailing wind. Whenever he noted cows with high respiration rates, he hosed them down then moved them to the small shed to alleviate their heat stress.

A panting score has been developed for feedlot beef cattle and this is fully described in Chapter 6.

6

Quantifying cow signals

This chapter provides scoring systems for many of the cow signals discussed in Chapter 5.

The main points of this chapter

- The body condition score provides a numerical assessment of the amount of muscle and fat covering the bones in the cow's hindquarters. It is based on a five point system for cows varying from poor condition to grossly overfat.
- The locomotion (or lameness) score provides a five point system to assess the ease with which cows can walk over a level surface. It varies from normal to severely lame.
- The hoof score provides a three point system to describe the degree of inflammation and infection of the hoof for each of three different hoof disease conditions.
- The leg score provides a three point system to assess the stance of the hind legs.
- The hygiene score provides a four point system to assess the degree of contamination of the hair and skin by dried and fresh dung on the udder and the lower hind leg regions.
- The rumen score provides a good measure of the cow's nutritional status using a five point system assessing rumen fill.
- The manure score assesses the visual composition and physical consistency of the dung using two different five point systems.

- The teat score assesses the teat health using a four point system.
- The panting score assesses respiration rate of heat stressed animals.

There are nine different scoring systems mentioned in Chapter 5 that provide many insights into cow health and wellbeing. These are fully described in this chapter and provide numerical values for:

- Body condition score: visual estimate of the amount of muscle and fat covering the bones of an animal
- Locomotion/lameness score: subjective assessment of how easily a cow walks on a level surface
- Hoof score: visual and descriptive assessment of the health of the hooves
- Leg score: the stance of the hindlegs
- Hygiene score: the contamination of manure and dirt on the udder and lower hind legs of cows
- Rumen score: the rumen fill as an indicator of the feed intake and rate of passage of feed over the last few hours
- Manure score: the visual composition and physical consistency of the faeces
- Teat score: the impact of the milking system on teat health
- Panting score: the impact of heat stress on the cow's wellbeing.

In addition to his book *Cow Signals: A Practical Guide For Dairy Farm Management* (Hulsen 2011), Hulsen (2013) has published a second book entitled *Cow Signals Checkbook: Working On Health, Production And Welfare* which provides a detailed series of checklists and instruction cards to help quantify various aspects of the cow and heifer's health and wellbeing. This new book contains many coloured pictures and diagrams highlighting the visual aspects of good dairy cow housing and management. Many of these pictorial standards are presented in this chapter (in black and white). An overview of the key checklists to assess cow health and welfare and also disease and distress are presented in Appendices 3 and 4 respectively.

6.1   Scoring body condition

Condition scoring is the visual evaluation of the amount of muscle and fat covering the bones of an animal. It can be assessed independently of live weight, gut fill and pregnancy status and involves observing specific points on the animal. Body condition affects milk production and reproductive performance. Scoring enables farmers to compare the condition of their cows with recommended targets. Knowledge of condition scoring then enables farmers to manage their feeding programs better.

The body condition is a very useful tool to monitor feeding management by providing a subjective estimate of the amount of muscle and subcutaneous fat between the pin bones and the tail head, over the hip and covering the lumbar vertebrae. Changes in condition take place over a matter of weeks or months. It increases when energy intake exceeds energy output and decreases when energy output exceeds energy intake.

For an overweight cow, there is a risk that around the time of calving and in early lactation, she will consume too little. A thin cow has poor immunity. Sharp falls in condition may lead to fertility problems and low resistance to disease. Fertility problems include cystic ovaries, inactive ovaries, poor non-existent heats and a poor corpus luteum.

Measuring standards have been developed to follow trends in body condition and to feed cows according to their energy requirements. Hulsen (2011) uses a five point scale where the senior author's previous books have used an eight point scale that was developed for the Victorian dairy industry; this is fully described in Chapter 18 of Moran (2005) which also discusses target condition scores at various stages during the lactation cycle and the frequency and best times to body condition your milking herd. Because the five point score is the preferred method in most Asian, European and US dairy management books, it will be used in this manual and is presented in Table 6.1 and Figure 6.1.

Target condition scores for cows and heifers are as follows:

Situation	Cows	Heifers
Pre-calving	2.5–3	2.5–3
Pre-service	2–3	2–2.5
Drying off	2.5–3	

If the average score is:

- within the normal range, the cows are receiving sufficient energy in their ration
- high, there is a risk that feed intake will be depressed at the beginning of the next lactation, so ensure cows are not too fat at the end of the current lactation
- low, energy intake has been insufficient and resistance to disease could be adversely affected, so increase feed intake and/or energy density of the ration.

If the spread of scores within the herd is:

- wide, there are big differences between cows in both energy intake and energy requirements, so determine how these large differences occurred and regroup cows according to their energy requirements
- narrow, the cows are all likely to be receiving sufficient energy.

Cows should be condition scored repeatedly to assist with feeding decisions. They can be interpreted as follows:

- if the score is within the normal range, then feeding management is correct
- if the score is below the normal range and changes by less than 0.75 points, then feeding management throughout lactation is correct but overall condition can be improved

Table 6.1. Descriptors for condition scoring of dairy cows for the 5 *(and 8 point)* scoring system.

5 point	8 point	Condition	Descriptors*
1	1–3	Very poor	Very thin Spine like teeth on a saw Transverse processes prominent with more than half the length visible Pin bones are very prominent, with a deep V shape cavity below the tail head and no fatty tissue under the skin
2	4, 5	Moderate	Skeleton clearly visible Individual vertebrae can be identified on the spine Transverse processes are 1/2 to 1/3 visible with the ends rounded and can be identified individually Pin bones are prominent with a U cavity below the tail head and some fat under skin
3	6	Good	Skeleton and covering are well balanced Spine forms a sharp ridge Transverse processes are 1/4 visible and individual vertebrae can still be identified but only by pressing on them Pin bones are rounded and smooth, with a shallow cavity below the tail head and fat cover over whole area, skin smooth, pelvis can be felt
4	7	Fat	There is excess fat covering Individual vertebrae cannot be identified Transverse processes have a smooth and rounded edge Pin bones are covered in fat with a shallow cavity below the tail head and patches of fat evident
5	8	Grossly fat or obese	Spine is covered with fat The ridge of transverse processes is barely visible Pin bones are completely covered in fat with the cavity filled with fat rolls The pelvis is impalpable, even with firm pressure

* The spine is assessed over the lumbar vertebrae; the transverse processes are the horizontal parts of the lumbar vertebrae; the pin bones are the bones on either side of the tail head.

- if the score decreases by more than 0.75 points during early lactation, then energy intake is too low hence dry cow, transition and early lactation feeding should all be reassessed
- if cows become over fat towards the end of lactation, then the energy:protein balance in the milking ration should be finetuned.

6.2 Locomotion and lameness scoring

Lameness is an increasing problem in both grazing and housed cows, and can often lead to serious economic implications. Locomotion scoring from 1 to 5 (for increasing lameness) provides a quick measure of the cow's ability to walk normally (Sprechter *et al.* 1997). The descriptors are presented in Table 6.2.

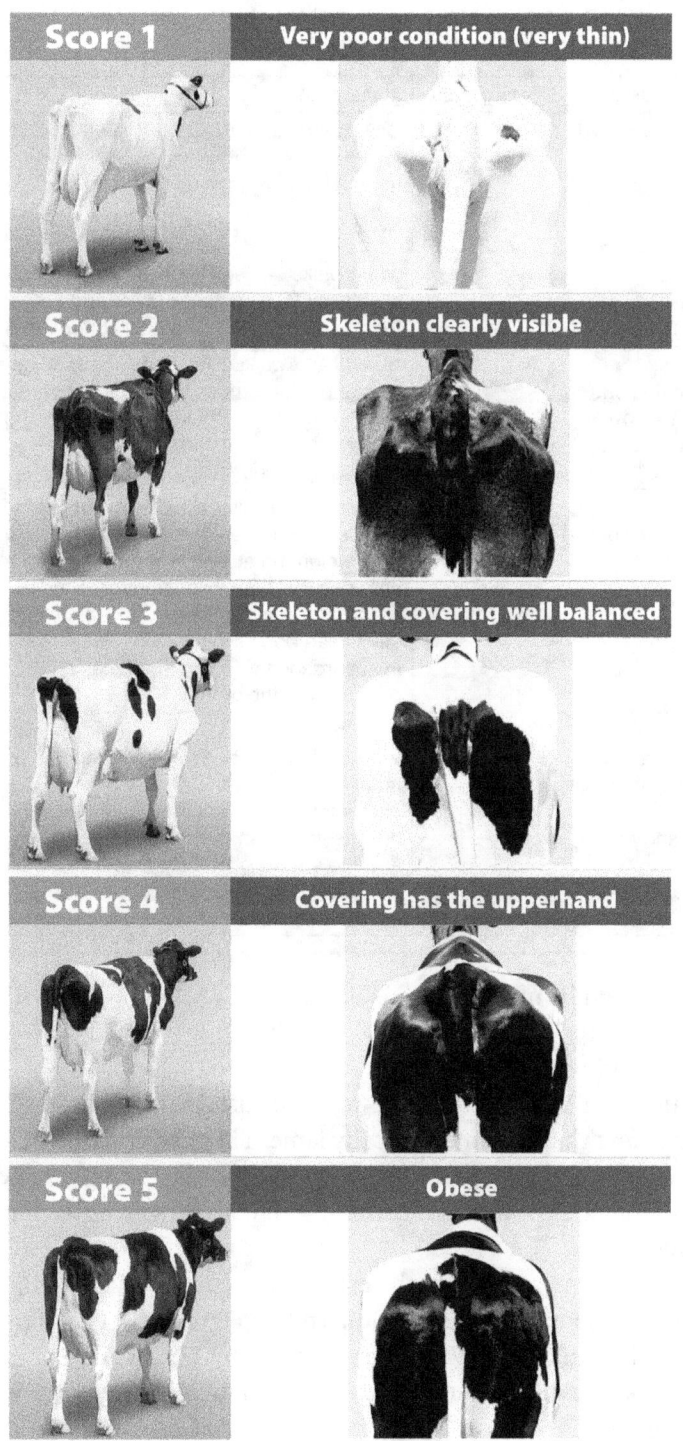

Figure 6.1: Pictorial standards of body condition scores in milking cows.

Table 6.2. Locomotion score guide based on observations of back posture, head and limb position and behaviour when walking.

Score	Clinical description	Back posture	Assessment	Decline
1	Smooth and fluid movement. *Normal.*	Flat	Cow stands and walks with a level back. All legs bear weight evenly. Joints flex freely. Head carriage remains steady as the animal moves. Gait is normal.	Feed: 0% Milk: 0%
2	Ability to move freely not diminished. *Mildly lame.*	Flat or arch	Cow stands with level back, but arches when walks. All legs bear weight. Joints slightly stiff. Head hangs lower and further from her body. Gait is slightly abnormal.	Feed: 1% Milk: 0%
3	Capable of locomotion but ability to move is compromised. *Moderately lame.*	Arch	Stands and walks with arched back. Slight limp and short strides in one or more legs. Joint shows signs of stiffness but does not impede freedom of movement. Head carriage remains steady.	Feed: 3% Milk: 5%
4	Ability to move freely is obviously diminished. *Lame.*	Arch	Arched back is always evident and gait is one deliberate step at a time. Reluctant to bear weight on at least one limp leg but still uses that limb in locomotion. Strides are hesitant and deliberate and joints are stiff. Head bobs slightly as animal moves in accordance with sore hoof making contact with the ground.	Feed: 7% Milk: 17%
5	Ability to move is severely restricted. Must be vigorously encouraged to stand and/or move. *Severely lame.*	3-legged	Extreme arched back when standing and walking. Inability to bear weight on one or more legs. Obvious joint stiffness characterised by lack of joint flexion with very hesitant and deliberate strides. One or more strides obviously shortened. Head obviously bobs as affected hoof makes contact with the ground.	Feed: 16% Milk: 36%

Observations should be made of cows standing and walking (gait), with emphasis on their back posture. The observation should be made on a flat surface that provides good footing.

Locomotion scores of individual cows can be used to select cows for hoof examination before they become clinically lame. Those with scores of 2 and 3 are considered subclinically lame and their hooves should be examined and trimmed to prevent more serious problems. Scores of 4 and 5 represent cows that are clinically lame.

The higher the lameness score, the greater the reduction in feed intake and milk yield and the poorer the body condition (see Figure 6.2). For example, a score of 4 can reduce DM intakes by 7% and milk yields by 17%, while a score of 5 can reduce DM intakes by 16% and milk yields by 36% (Sprechter *et al.* 1997). Advice should be sought if more than 3% of first-calving cows, or more than 2% of older cows, show signs of lameness.

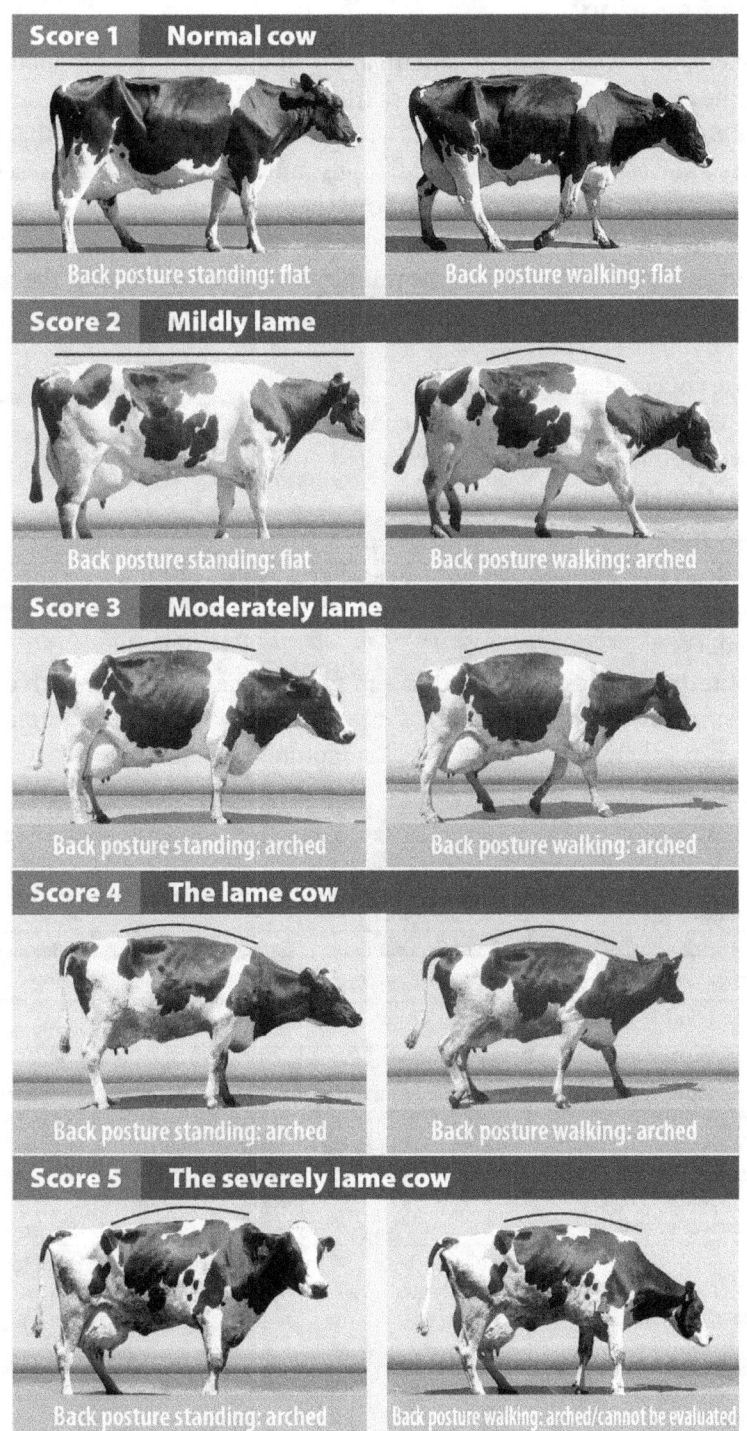

Figure 6.2: Pictorial standards of locomotion scores in milking cows.

6.3 Hoof scoring

Hoof problems can cause cows great pain and will directly affect production because lame cows visit feeding areas less frequently. It is important to detect symptoms early. Hulsen (2011) presents a 3 point hoof scoring system that can incorporate a variety of symptoms occurring simultaneously. This is presented in Table 6.3 and Figure 6.3a. The positioning of the hoof problems and their degree of intensity in the Figure is the same as in Table 6.3 with foul-in-the-foot as the top three pictures, digital dermatitis as the middle three and laminitis as the bottom three pictures in Figure 6.3a.

Other causes of cow lameness

Hulsen (2011) describes six other hoof conditions but without scoring systems for their degrees of intensity. These are presented pictorially in Figure 6.3b.

The top three pictures are:

- **Healthy hoof:** the hoof wall and the entire sole are weight bearing.
- **Solar ulcer:** inflammatory lesions in sole area which occur as a result of either laminitis or bruising to the sole (or both). Soft hooves are more likely to be affected.
- **Combination of digital dermatitis and foul-in-the-foot:** these both occur under similar conditions, namely, wet feet and dirty floors. They often occur together in which case the cow shows symptoms of both.

Table 6.3. Descriptors of three hoof problems at varying degrees of intensity (or scores) (see also Figure 6.3a).

Disease condition	1	2	3
Foul-in-the-foot C: Bacterial infection T: Foot trimming, formalin footbaths* P: same as T, dry floors	Mild inflammation of skin with yellow putrid discharge between claws	Severe inflammation of skin which affects heels (cracks, punctures)	Extensive moist inflammation of heels extending into inter-digital space
Digital dermatitis or strawberry footrot C: Bacterial infection T: Foot trimming, antibiotic spray, bandage for 3 days P: reduce level of infection	Round discrete lesion causing pain (in a healing or mild case)	Slight deterioration of hoof tissue at coronary band. Painful and bleeds easily	Large strawberry-like extremely sore lesion. Bleeds easily
Laminitis C: physical trauma T: anti-inflammatories, soft surfaces P: adequate fibre in diet, good stall design, correct/remove housing problems	Small localised discolouration	Discolouration of about one-third of sole	Discolouration of almost entire sole

Abbreviations: C, cause; T, treatment; P, prevention.
*Formalin footbaths have 4 L formaldehyde per 100 L water.

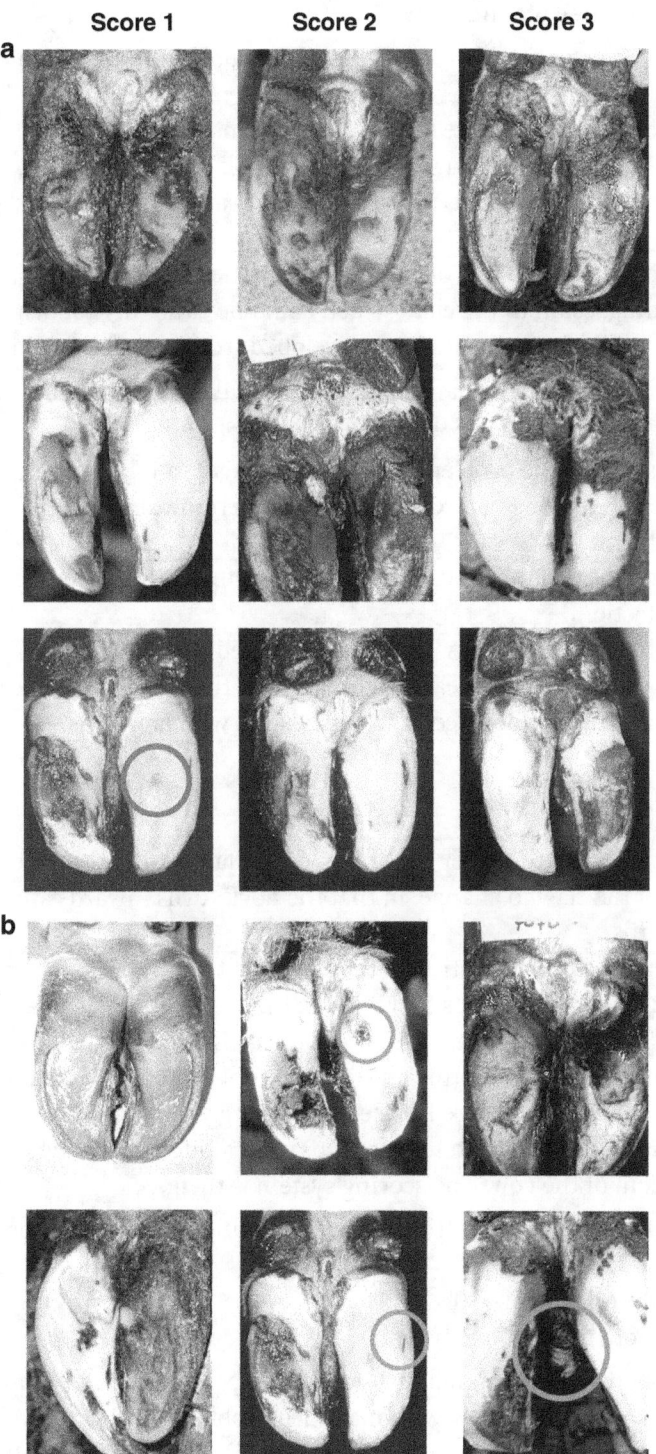

Figure 6.3: a) Pictorial standards of hoof score in dairy cattle. b) Other causes of lameness in dairy cattle.

The bottom three pictures are:

- **False sole:** false or double sole occurs after acute laminitis or radical dietary changes. In many cases there are few other signs of laminitis.
- **White line disease:** a white (or pink) line forms between the sole and the wall and white line disease occurs if there is a break in the continuity. There can be both mild and severe forms. Most important causes are laminitis and trauma (bruising).
- **Interdigital growths:** this occurs between the claws and develops because of a longstanding lesion in the cleft, which could be either digital dermatitis or foul-in-the-foot. The lesion could have developed from an infection in the cleft.

Hoof lesions are signals that can be used to make improvements in herd management with a rough classification as follows:

- Laminitis: metabolic problems, errors or changes in ration formulation and amount offered, housing problems such as overcrowding, slippery floors and poor stalls.
- Digital dermatitis: infectious diseases, associated with low resistance and high risk of infection.
- Foul-in-the-foot: infectious diseases, associated with high risk of infection.
- Solar ulcers: white line disease, trauma, when the herd is unsettled and/or slippery or uneven floors, could be associated with laminitis.

6.4 Leg scoring

With foul-in-the-foot, the outer claw often grows faster than the inner claw causing the position of the claw to change, in that the hock turns inwards and the claw rotates outwards.

Leg scoring is a quantification of the stance of the hindlegs (Figure 6.4). It is related to the height differences between the inner and outer claws and the way the cow places her foot. Cows rotate their feet outwards to relieve painful areas in the sole and are more likely to do this on slippery floors when they walk with more weight on their heels. The score is based on the degrees rotation from perpendicular (90°) when both legs point parallel along the backbone from the back to the front of the cow. The scoring system is then:

- **Score 1:** 0° to 17° from 90°; this is the ideal situation although hoof problems can still occur
- **Score 2:** 17° to 24° from 90°
- **Score 3:** more than 24° from 90°.

Figure 6.4 presents diagrams of hindleg stances and a leg score calculator. It also includes a picture of a cow with major leg problems in that the right foot is virtually parallel with the spine (Score 1) but the left leg is turned outwards, swollen and painful. This is a score 3 requiring immediate attention and treatment.

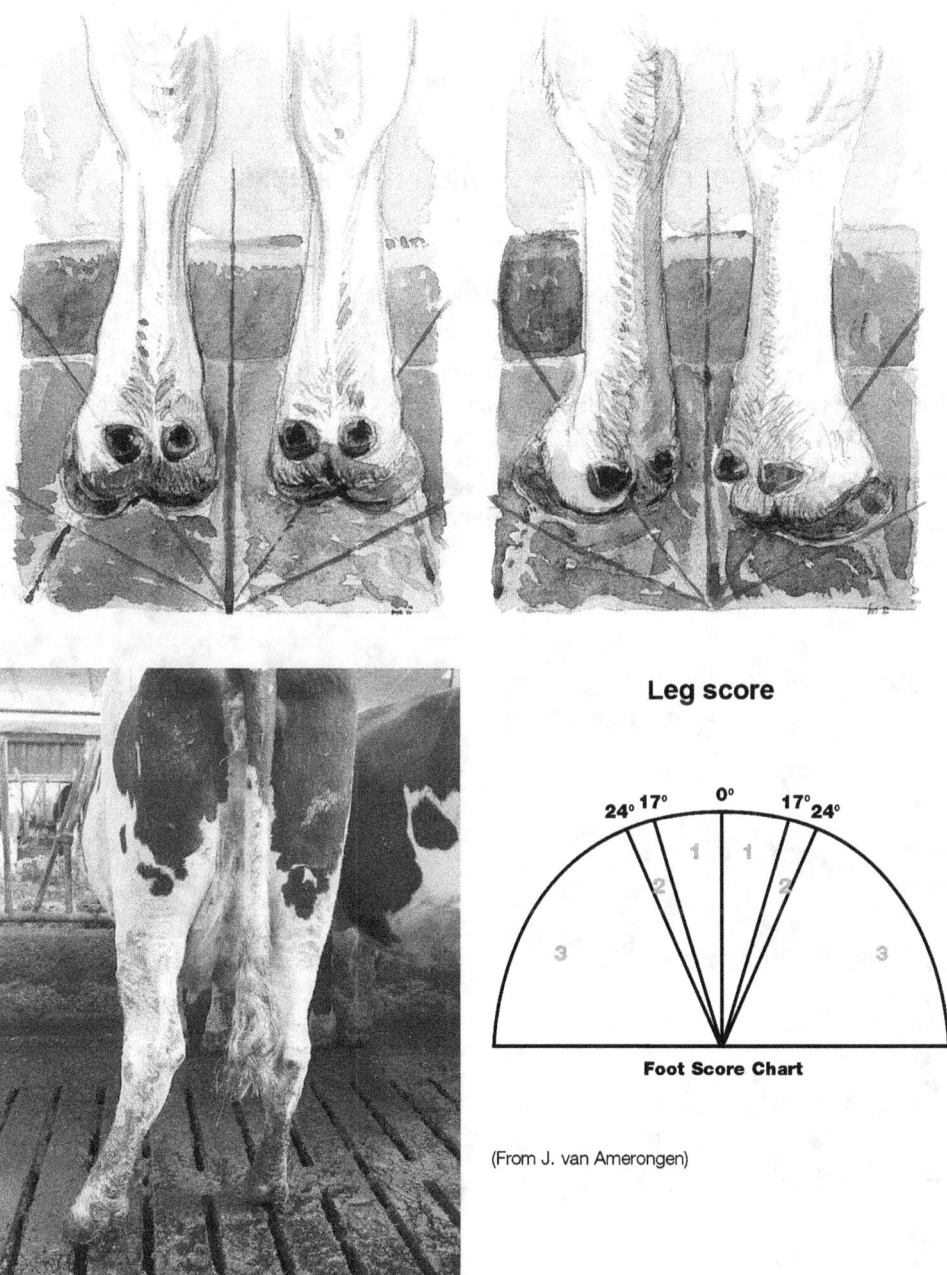

Figure 6.4: Pictorial standards of leg scores in milking cows.

If there are high proportions of cows with Scores 2 or 3, the technique and frequency of foot trimming should be re-evaluated as well as other factors affecting leg stance.

6.5 Scoring cow hygiene and shed cleanliness

The amount of dried and fresh manure on the cow gives an idea of the level of hygiene on the farm. The dirtier the cows, the higher the chance of udder and skin infections. A decrease of one point in the herd hygiene score equates to an increase of 50 000 cells/ml in milk bulk somatic cell count. The presence of dirty cows also indicates other management factors to assess such as ventilation, nutrition, stall dimensions and cleanliness of the laneways.

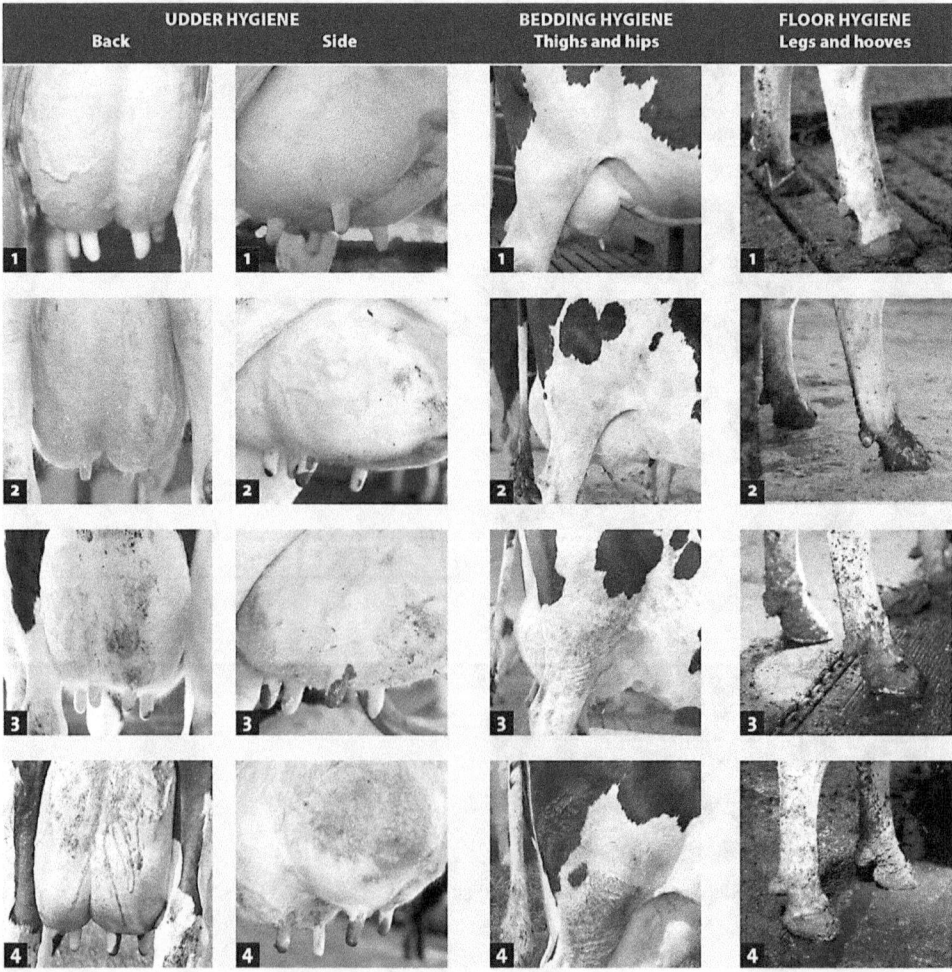

Figure 6.5: Pictorial standards of hygiene scores in milking cows.

There are three separate areas to score cow hygiene, namely, the udder (the back and the side), the abdomen and upper legs (thighs and hips) and the lower legs (legs and hooves). Individual scores are not important, just the herd average. When scoring a herd of cows, place a tick in the appropriate box for each score, then calculate the percentage of cows with each hygiene score. The scoring is very subjective using the pictures standards in Figure 6.5 to score from 1 (very clean) through to 4 (unacceptable).

As a guide to an acceptable level of cow hygiene on a well managed farm:

Udder hygiene: only 10% of the cows score 3 or 4

Thigh hygiene: only 15% of the cows score 3 or 4

Lower leg and hooves hygiene: only 20% of the cows score 3 or 4.

How clean are the udders and teats when the cow enters the milking parlour? Udder hygiene is influenced by stall cleanliness, amount and type of bedding material, cleanliness of alleyways, clipping of udders, comfort in the stall, manure consistency and health of the herd.

How clean are the stalls? Thigh hygiene is influenced by stall care and bedding, cow comfort in the stall, manure consistency and health of the herd.

How clean are the alleyways? Leg and hoof hygiene is influenced by alleyway cleaning, cleaning the holding yard for milking the cows and space allowance per cow.

6.6 Rumen scoring

Hulsen (2011) considers rumen fill as a good indicator of the nutritional status of the animal. It quantifies the intake of feed and its rate of passage of feed over the previous few hours. The rumen fill depends on a combination of:

- the quantity of feed consumed
- its rate of digestion and passage from the rumen to the abomasum and the lower gut.

The rates of digestion and passage of the feed depend on the dietary components (whether they are rapidly or slowly degraded in the rumen), its particle size when fed and the balance of dietary nutrients. It must be remembered that after 5 months pregnancy, the developing uterus visibly occupies some of the abdominal cavity. The scoring is conducted on the left flank of the cow and is presented in Table 6.4 and Figures 6.6a and 6.6b. The rumen score is assessed by observing the area between the ribs at the front, the vertebrae at the top and hook bone at the back, as indicated in drawing in Figure 6.6b.

Score all animals during the day or whenever convenient. As a rumen score is just a snapshot, it is best to score animals at different times of the day to get a good overall impression of their rumen fill. The ideal rumen scores vary for different

Table 6.4. Descriptors used to quantify rumen scores and their diagnoses.

Score	Descriptor	Diagnosis
1	A deep dip in the left flank The skin under the lumbar vertebrae curves inwards The skin fold from the hook bone goes vertically downwards The para lumbar fossa behind the last rib is more than one hand width deep Viewed from the side, this part of the flank has a rectangular appearance	The cow has eaten little or nothing which could be due to sudden illness or insufficient or unpalatable feed
2	The skin under the lumbar vertebrae curves inwards The skin fold from the hook bone runs diagonally forward towards the last rib The para lumbar fossa behind the last rib is one hand width deep Viewed from the side, this part of the flank has a triangular appearance	This score is often seen in cows in the first week after calving Later in lactation, this is a sign of insufficient feed intake or a too high rate of passage
3	The skin under the lumbar vertebrae goes vertically down for one hand width and then curves outward. The skin fold from the hook bone is not visible The para lumbar fossa behind the last rib is still just visible	This is the right score for milking cows with a good feed intake and when the feed remains in the rumen for the optimal time
4	The skin under the lumbar vertebrae curves outwards No para lumber fossa is visible behind the last rib	This is the correct score for cows nearing the end of lactation and for dry cows
5	The lumbar vertebrae are not visible as the rumen is well filled The skin over the whole belly is quite tight There is no visible transition between the flank and ribs	This is the correct score for dry cows

classes of stock, with the target for lactating cows being 3.0 and the target for dry cows being 4.0. This is because the heavily pregnant uterus alone in dry cows would lead to higher scores. Throughout the day, rumen scores should only be 0.5 above or 0.5 below these targets. The optimal rumen score for rations with low rates of passage (high fibrous diets) would be higher than for a ration with fast rate of passage (high concentrate diets).

Specific animals with low rumen scores should be monitored more closely, while high variation within the herd requires diagnosis and eliminating the causes. If the overall score is too low or too high, feed intake and composition should be monitored.

6.7 Manure scoring

Manure (or dung as it is often called) is a mirror of the digestive tract. By closely assessing the manure, you get an indication of the balance of the ration. You need to pay attention to consistency and the level of digestion. Consistency relates to the

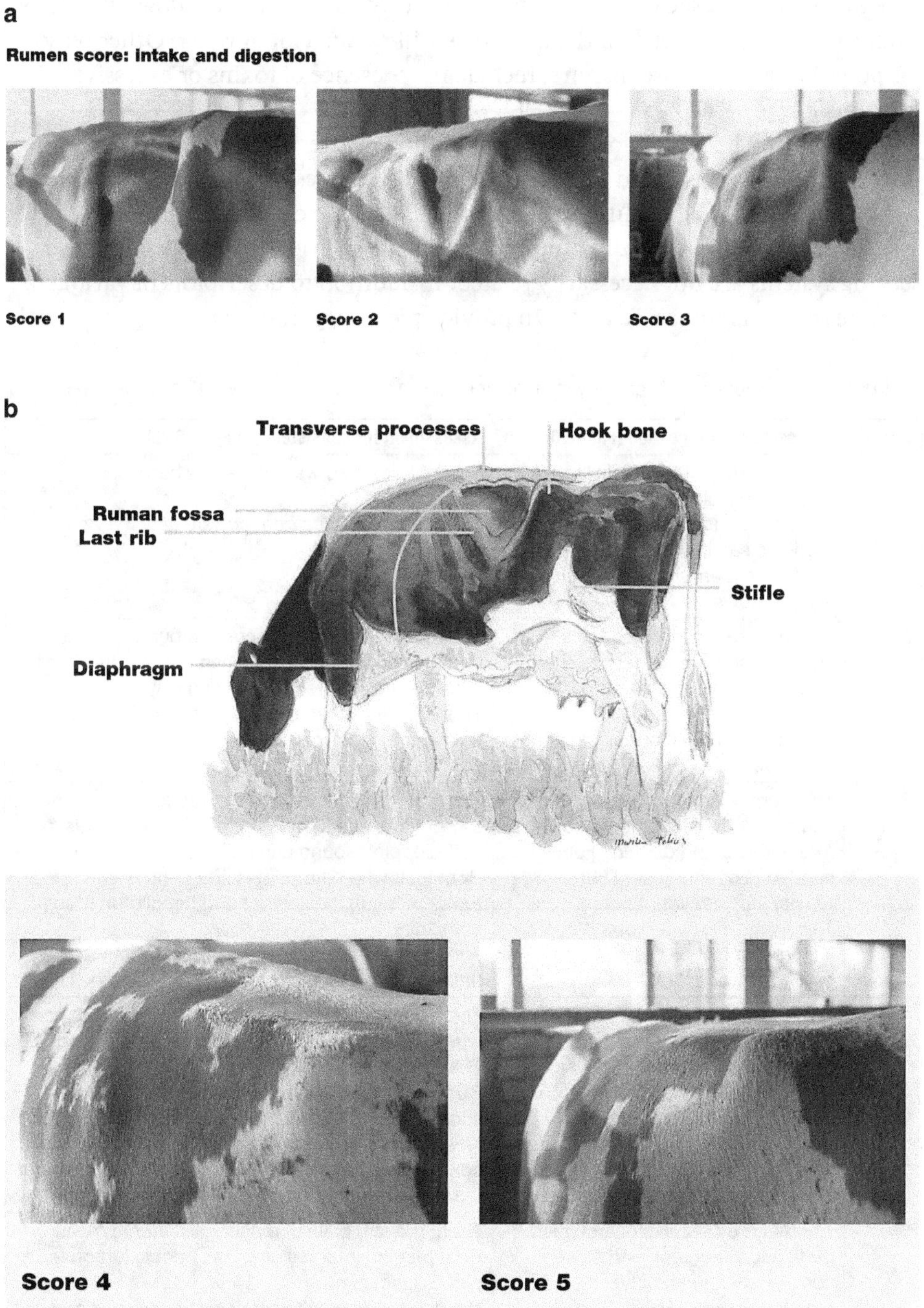

a

Rumen score: intake and digestion

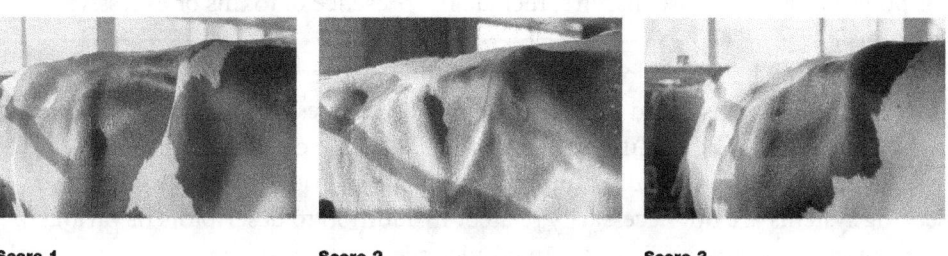

Score 1   Score 2   Score 3

b

Transverse processes   Hook bone

Ruman fossa
Last rib

Stifle

Diaphragm

Score 4   Score 5

Figure 6.6: a) Pictorial standards of rumen scores 1, 2 and 3 in milking cows. b) Pictorial standards of rumen scores 4 and 5 in milking cows.

moisture content of the manure. If there are lots of abnormal breakdown products from the feed, the contents of the intestines will retain a lot of water. Other reasons for poor digestion – loose manure, include the presence of toxins or excessive minerals in the diet.

Manure can be scored for digestion and for consistency as shown in Table 6.5. The digestion score is based on taking a close look at fresh dung that has just been passed and feeling the manure with a gloved hand. The consistency score is assessed by eye and by treading into the manure with your gumboot. These two scoring systems are not necessarily related. In addition to descriptors of various manure scores, Figures 6.7a and 6.7b provide pictorial standards.

Table 6.5. Descriptors used to quantify manure for digestion and for consistency with *diagnoses in italics.*

Score	Assessment for digestion (Figure 6.7a)	Assessment for consistency (Figure 6.7b)
1	The manure glistens, feels like a creamy emulsion and is homogeneous. No undigested feed particles can be felt or seen. *This is the ideal score for milking and dry cows.*	The manure is so watery that it's barely recognisable. *This manure comes from cows that are very ill.*
2	The manure glistens and feels smooth and homogeneous. There are a few undigested feed particles that can be seen and felt. *This is acceptable for milking and dry cows.*	The manure is like a thin custard but is recognisable as manure. When it lands on a hard surface, the splatter goes a long way *This happens when grazing young, rich grass and when there is an imbalance in the ration.*
3	The manure appears slightly dull and does not feel homogeneous. After closing and opening your hand, bits of undigested fibre remain stuck to your fingers. *This manure is acceptable for in-calf heifers and dry cows but not for milking cows.*	The manure is like a thick custard forming a cowpat to a height of 2 to 3 cm. When it lands, a soft plopping sound can be heard. Boot test: when the boot is lifted, there is a footprint left in the cowpat and the manure does not stick. *This is an ideal consistency for manure as the ration is visibly well digested.*
4	The manure is dull in appearance and contains some coarse undigested feed particles, which are clearly visible. After closing and opening your hand, a ball of undigested feed remains in your hand. *The ration needs to be adjusted.*	The manure is thick, makes a heavy plopping noise when landing, is well formed and stacks in rings. The height is a finger's length or more. Boot test: when the boot is lifted, the manure sticks to it and a boot print is left behind. *This indicates an imbalance in the ration. For dry cows and in calf heifers this may be acceptable but the ration formulation should still be checked.*
5	The manure contains coarse feed particles and undigested ration components are clearly recognisable. *The ration needs adjusting.*	There are stiff balls of manure, like horse manure. Boot test: an impression of the boot is left on top of the dung. *Dry cows and in calf heifers often pass this sort of manure and it indicates the ration formulation should be checked. Check individual cows for disease (such as ketosis).*

a Manure Score A: Looking and feeling for the level of digestion of fresh manure

This scoring method is based on taking a close look at fresh manure that has just been
passed, and feeling the manure with your hand

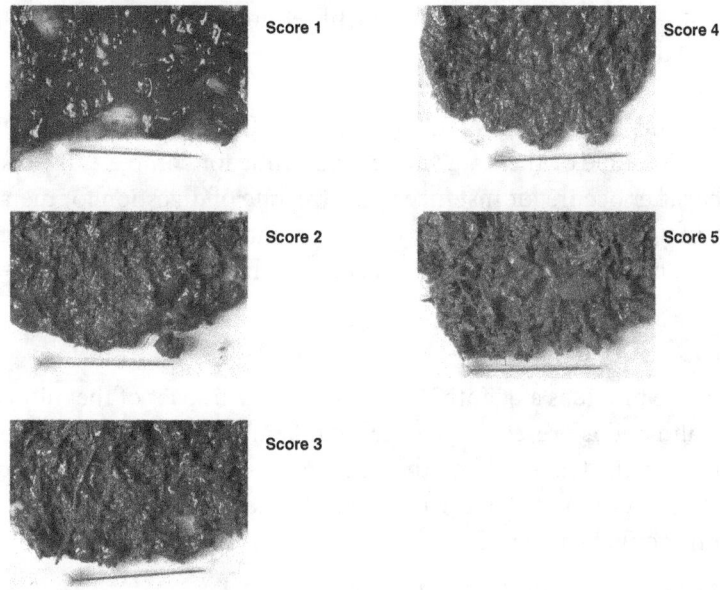

b Manure Score B: consistency of fresh cow manure

The scoring of fresh manure is done in two different ways: by eye and by
treading your boot in the manure

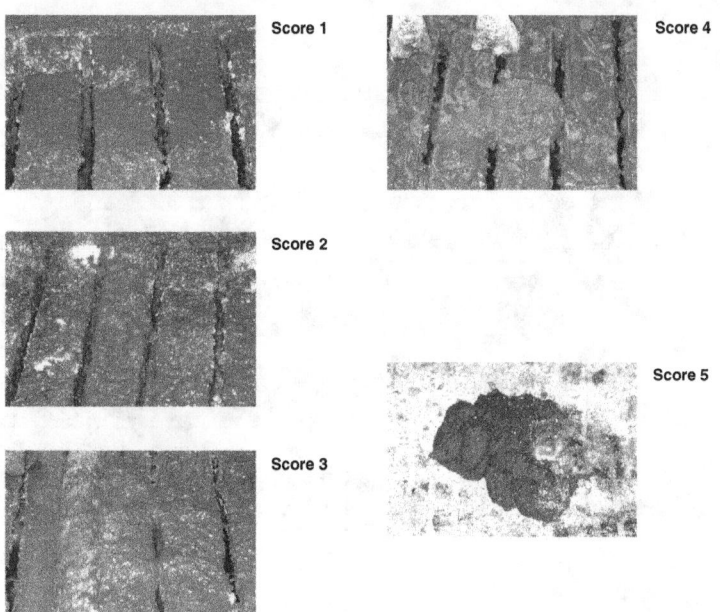

Figure 6.7: a) Pictorial standards for scoring manure for digestion in milking cows. b) Pictorial standards for scoring manure for consistency in milking cows.

The residue in a sieve after rinsing the manure with water provides a good indication of how well the feed has been digested and how much the cow is ruminating. Less than half the manure should remain in the sieve, while all the grain should have been digested and the fibre should show signs of having been chewed and digested.

When evaluating digestion you are looking for bits of undigested feed. Ideally every component of the diet should be digested. If parts are not digested, either they are indigestible or there was not enough time for complete digestion to take place. The latter occurs for instance when the rate of digestion for dietary energy and protein are not balanced, due to incorrect ration formulation. From the time feed is eaten until it is passed in the faeces takes between 36 and 72 h.

6.8 Teat scoring

The teat score provides a quantitative guide on the impact of the milking system on teat health and is presented pictorially in Figure 6.8 then described in Table 6.6. It assesses both the teat ends and the skin around the teat. Cows should be scored immediately after removal of the milk cluster and it should be conducted monthly.

Action should be taken if:

- more than 20% of the cows have scores of 3 or 4
- more than 30% of the cows between the second and fifth month of lactation have scores of 3 or 4
- when the overall score is considerably worse than the previous scoring.

Teat score

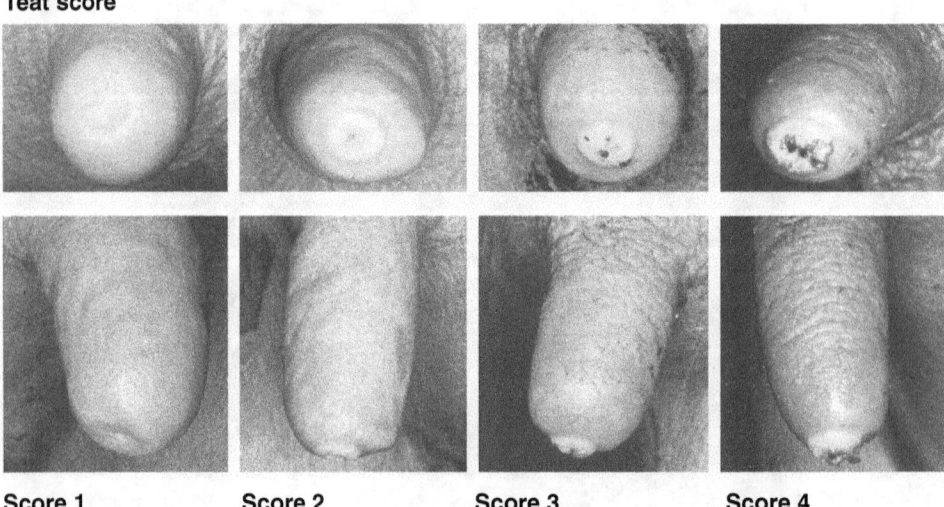

Score 1   Score 2   Score 3   Score 4

Figure 6.8: Pictorial standards for teat scoring in milking cows.

Table 6.6. Descriptors used to score teat health.

Score	Descriptor
1	No calluses
2	Smooth fairly thick callused ring around teat end
3	Moderately rough callused ring, with some fraying around the edges
4	Very rough calloused ring with a lot of fraying

6.9 Panting score

The Australian beef industry developed a panting score for use with feedlot beef cattle (Meat and Livestock Australia 2006). This could also be useful to dairy farmers to assess heat stress in milking cows. Table 6.7 summarises the key features of the panting score.

Guidelines for lofted beef cattle are as follows:

- If more than 10% of the cattle exhibit panting scores of 2 or more, cattle handling should cease and only resume when conditions become cooler and cattle have returned to normal.
- Cattle with panting scores of 3.5 or more are in danger of death.
- If more than 10% of the cattle exhibit panting scores of 3.5 or more, there is potential for a serious problem to develop unless measures are taken to cool the stock.
- The transition from 2.5 to 4.5 can happen quickly, in less than 2 h, under extreme conditions.

Table 6.7. Panting score to quantify heat stress.

Panting score	Breaths/minute	Breathing condition
0	< 40	Normal with no panting. Difficult to see chest movement.
1	40–70	Slight panting, mouth closed with no salivation. Easy to see chest movement.
2	70–120	Fast panting with salivation present. No open mouth panting.
2.5	70–120	As for 2 but with occasional open mouth panting. Tongue not extended.
3	120–160	Open mouth panting and some drooling. Neck extended and head usually up.
3.5	120–160	As for 3 but with tongue out slightly, occasionally fully extended for short periods and excessive drooling.
4	> 160	Open mouth with tongue fully extended for prolonged periods and excessive drooling.
4.5	Variable	As for 4 but head down. Cattle breathe from flank. Drooling may cease.

The panting score was developed primarily for lot-fed beef cattle often kept outside in dirt yards with or without access to shade. This is not the normal situation with milking cows which are either grazing at pasture (where heat loads are not as extreme as in dirt yards) or are maintained in sheds. Furthermore, the type of heat load is often different. In Australia, feedlot beef cattle are usually maintained in dry regions with high solar heat loads, whereas Asian dairy cows are usually kept in sheds where the heat load is more from high humidity and air movement can be poor. However, there are some dairy regions in Asia, such as Punjab in Pakistan where dairy cows are subjected to similar types of environmental management and heat stress as Australian lofted beef cattle.

7

Cow comfort

This chapter discusses cow comfort, what it is and how it is influenced by shed design and other physical facilities on the farm.

The main points of this chapter

- There are various definitions of cow comfort and these range from the cow's comfort zone or zone of thermoneutrality, to their physical environment or ability to do what they want to do and when they want to do it. The most complete definition is the cow's overall wellbeing that takes into account their psychological as well as physiological needs.
- A comfortable cow is then 'at peace' with her perception of the world.
- Cow comfort for walking, standing, exercise and lying are the keys for healthy and mobile cows and studies have shown that up to 20% of the cow's potential is determined by how comfortable she is and whether her demands are met.
- Daily time budgets for productive milking cows should allow for 12 to 14 h resting, including at least 6 h rumination, 5 to 6 h eating with 9 to 14 meals per day and 2 to 3 h standing and walking in alleys.
- To achieve cow wellbeing, farmers must address the twin issues of housing and management, where management covers all the normal farm practices associated with dairy farming. Ideally, the farm's physical facilities should be optimised before putting the cows in the shed.
- One of the most controversial aspects when confining cows to a shed is the type of stalls they are provided with. Tie stalls are the most common

in Asia – they are purely for the convenience of the farmer. In more developed dairy industries free stalls are the most common for shedded cows, because cow comfort is given a higher priority (and this results in higher yields).

- With tie stall systems, each cow is restrained in a separate stall. Tie stalls restrict normal behaviour and the opportunity for social contact. They limit the ability for each cow to self-groom, and all too commonly are associated with poor hygiene and uncomfortable lying surfaces. Boredom and frustration often lead to abnormal stereotype behaviours.
- Tie stalls are *not* appropriate for the optimum wellbeing of milking cows and these conditions can negatively affect milk yields and cow longevity.
- When well-designed and managed, free stalls provide the ideal system for intensively managing dairy cows off pasture as each animal is provided with a specific place to rest, their management (feeding, cleaning and relaxing) is potentially optimised and the system can operate efficiently with minimal labour.
- Stall dimensions (to match cow size), the base material, type of bedding and manure management are the key factors in optimising stall usage.
- Other important facilities to incorporate into cowsheds include fans and sprinklers, hospital and isolation pens for sick animals, calving down pens, bull holding and mating pens, cattle race and crush and footbaths.
- For larger-scale dairy farms, cow comfort can be improved with rotating cow brushes, automatic cow showers and self-locking gates.
- This chapter concludes with plans and pictures of two 'animal friendly' small holder cow sheds.

The challenge for modern dairy production is the maintenance of healthy, long living cows with a high level of performance. As cows produce more milk, they become more sensitive to their environment. If we succeed in transferring the natural conditions into the cowshed, which means adapting the cowshed to the animal and not vice versa, this is a step towards more profitable dairy production with healthier animals.

7.1 Introduction

7.1.1 What is cow comfort?

There are several definitions of cow comfort.

- To many people, cow comfort simply refers to the climatic environment or the 'comfort zone'. This is the zone of a cow's thermoneutrality and is defined as the range in ambient temperature in which there are no measurable fluctuations in the cow's physiological processes. In this situation the energy input to output shows good biological efficiency with all the body processes functioning in their expected ranges. For the milking Friesian cow, this occurs between 6 and 18°C.

- Others consider comfort to be more related to the cow's physical environment, or their ability to do what they want to do and when they want to do it. In particular, it should allow cows to have their 12 to 14 h rest each day, undisturbed by other stock and in comfortable stalls or other resting spaces.
- Cow comfort should also take into account their appetites for both water and feed. With regard to feed, it should satisfy the requirements for their current levels of production (both milk and if pregnant, the needs of the growing foetus) but its nutritive quality, within reason, need not be taken into consideration. With regard to drinking water, ideally cows should be provided with a continuous supply of clean, fresh, quality water.
- It is generally agreed that cow comfort should also be extended to the cow's overall wellbeing, this means covering their psychological as well as physiological needs. Cows should not be continually fearful, which (as described by Klindworth *et al.* (2003) in Chapter 4) is their natural response to real or perceived threats, and serves to protect them from danger.
- Therefore, the complete definition of cow comfort addresses climatic stress, poorly designed and constructed housing, stock facilities and the potential behavioural stress from herd mates and stock people. It could simply be defined as a cow being 'at peace' with her perception of the world.

A comfortable cow is one that is at peace with her environment, and therefore should respond well to more intensive feeding and herd management. As a cow's appetite should not be limiting, any resultant higher feed nutrient intakes should produce more milk and achieve the positive energy balance required to conceive her next calf. The simplest assessment of cow comfort is her potential appetite, in that, generally speaking, if she is offered more she will eat it. As the marginal efficiency of utilising additional feed nutrients to synthesise animal products all too often decreases with increasing intake (Moran 2005), cow comfort cannot really be defined in terms of production response to any extra feed.

7.1.2 Physical cow comfort

Taking into account whether or not a cow feels comfortable walking, standing, exercising and lying down is vital for healthy and mobile cows and studies have shown that up to 20% of the cow's potential is determined by their demands on comfort. With well-designed laneways and resting stalls, supportive lying surfaces and non-slip walking surfaces, cows suffer less lameness, can behave more naturally and experience less stress, and therefore have higher milk yields and longer valuable lives.

Walking

The hoof structure allows the blood flow in the claw to work like a sponge. Load presses the blood out of the tissue and when the pressure is released, blood (hence the supply of nutrients to the claw) re-enters the tissue. As the anatomy of the cattle claw is ideally designed for soft floors, the activity of cows' hooves doubles when on soft floors compared to concrete. Less movement on a hard surface can result in reduced blood flow to the hoof which then results in inferior hoof horn quality. In addition, cows are more likely to allow bulls to mount them on soft rubber compared to concrete, this means they have a shorter time to first breeding and fewer days open.

Standing

Unlike when at grazing, where cows are continually moving and thus redistributing their weight on each foot, cows are forced to stand still while feeding in the shed. In addition, cows stand in laneways, in their stalls and in the collecting yard while waiting to be milked. Cows need to be able to stand undisturbed such as when stretching after a period of lying down or if they prefer to ruminate standing up.

Exercise

Exercise decreases the incidence of leg problems, mastitis, bloat and for young stock, calf-related disorders. Outdoor exercise improves bovine health and wellbeing regardless of tie stall or free stall housing. Free stall housed cows with outdoor exercise have better claw health, suffer less from lameness, tarsal joint lesions, teat injuries and require fewer medical treatments. Providing a portion of the daily ration in an outdoor exercise area effectively doubles the amount of time cows can spend outdoors. Even small amounts of exercise can improve fitness via reductions in heart rate and plasma lactate levels. The rate of detection and the duration of oestrus are higher for cows on dirt yards or pasture than they are for cows on concrete.

Surface

A good surface provides even pressure distribution and good grip. On such a surface, cows take large strides, where their hind hoof steps into the print of their front hoof and their hooves rotate correctly while walking. On a good surface, animals do not slip easily and this makes them more peaceful and confident. They know that they can fight and flee safely. Being on a non-slip surface means that the cows more readily show signs when they are in oestrus. Their feed and water intakes will be better, as will their visits to the feed trough, stalls and to the milking area. They have less trouble with chronic hoof problems.

Lying

Cows should rest for 12 to 14 h per day in natural long lying bouts. It gives the hoofs a chance to dry out, which suppresses infections. Resting cows are out of the way, giving other cows more space to get to feed. Reduced total lying time or elongated lying periods are signs of inadequate lying comfort. Softer lying material (thick mattresses v thin mattresses and concrete) increases both lying time and milk yield. Cows that are lame have excessive lying times (> 14.5 h) and elongated lying bouts (> 90 min per bout).

Tethering

Tethering restricts the time cattle spend lying down for the first few weeks, when they display more intention movements but few actual bouts of lying. In the long term, the time spent lying may increase with tethering due to the forced inactivity. Compared to free stall and loose housing, stress levels are increased by tethering. The increased lying time is likely to stress the joints of tethered cattle and a significant proportion show swollen joints. Cubicle systems for loose housing are less damaging to cattle welfare than tethering systems, but the time that cows spend lying in cubicles is still less than in pens with deep straw bedding. High stocking rates of loose cows in straw yards or open yards should be avoided as they prevent cattle both synchronising their lying behaviour and lying for their preferred time.

Cows seek their own level of comfort and they should be provided with a relatively clean dry area in which to lie down. It should be conducive for cows to lie for as many hours of the day as they desire. There should be enough stalls or space so cows do not have to wait when they want to lie down. For every hour resting above 7 h, cows can produce up to an extra 1 kg milk. Blood flow to the udder, which is related to the level of milk production, is substantially higher (20 to 30%) when cows are lying down than when they are standing.

A daily time budget for a typical milking cow in a free stall shed in the US is:

- Eating: 5.5 h/day with 9 to 14 meals/day
- Resting: 12 to 14 h/day, including 6 h rumination
- Standing or walking in alleys: 2 to 3 h/day, which includes grooming, rumination, socialising and other activities
- Drinking: 0.5 h/day
- Total time needed: 21 to 22 h/day.

This indicates that cows have little time to spare, so time away from the pen should be minimised and this includes visiting the milking parlour generally twice daily.

Heat stress affects cow comfort and productivity. Milk production during hot weather can be improved by installing sunshades, sprinklers and fans, as well as by dietary modifications. Within temperate dairy breeds, Jersey and Brown Swiss tolerate heat stress better than Friesians. In one free stall shed in Indiana, in which sprinklers and fans were activated at 21°C, cooled cows produced 36 L/day of milk compared to only 32 L/day in uncooled cows.

7.1.3 Building for the cow

It is essential that when designing housing systems, farmers keep the following key principles in mind:

- To achieve cow productivity, farmers must address the twin issues of cow comfort and health, where health is the freedom from infections, injuries and metabolic problems.
- To achieve cow wellbeing, farmers must address the twin issues of housing and management, where management covers all the normal farm practices associated with dairy farming.
- Addressing cow comfort and housing means that the farm's physical facilities must be optimised before putting cows in sheds.

Cows grazing in a paddock have access to forage matter virtually all the time and to concentrates at least twice per day, at milking. These feeding goals should also be the aim when cows are maintained in sheds. They should be encouraged to make at least 12 trips each day from their place of rest to the feed and water troughs. This will only occur if cows 'feel good', have healthy legs and feet, and the route is safe and comfortable.

There are six key housing aspects of cow health and wellbeing, namely:

1. Access to clean, palatable water at least 21 h/d
2. Light with at least 6 h/d of darkness
3. Fresh and clean air
4. Rest, with a dry and comfortable place to lie down for at least 12 h/d
5. Space so cows can walk to feed and water troughs from their free stalls without fear
6. Palatable and well formulated feed, on offer for at least 21 h/d.

The remainder of this chapter discusses the physical aspects of ensuring cow comfort. Details of housing systems have been presented in a previous book (in Chapter 13 of Moran 2012a) so this chapter will concentrate on the stock welfare aspects of cow housing and present some examples of 'animal friendly' small holder cowsheds.

7.2 Stalls for shedded cows

One of the most controversial aspects when confining cows to a shed is the type of stalls they are provided with (see Figure 7.1). Tie stalls are the most common in

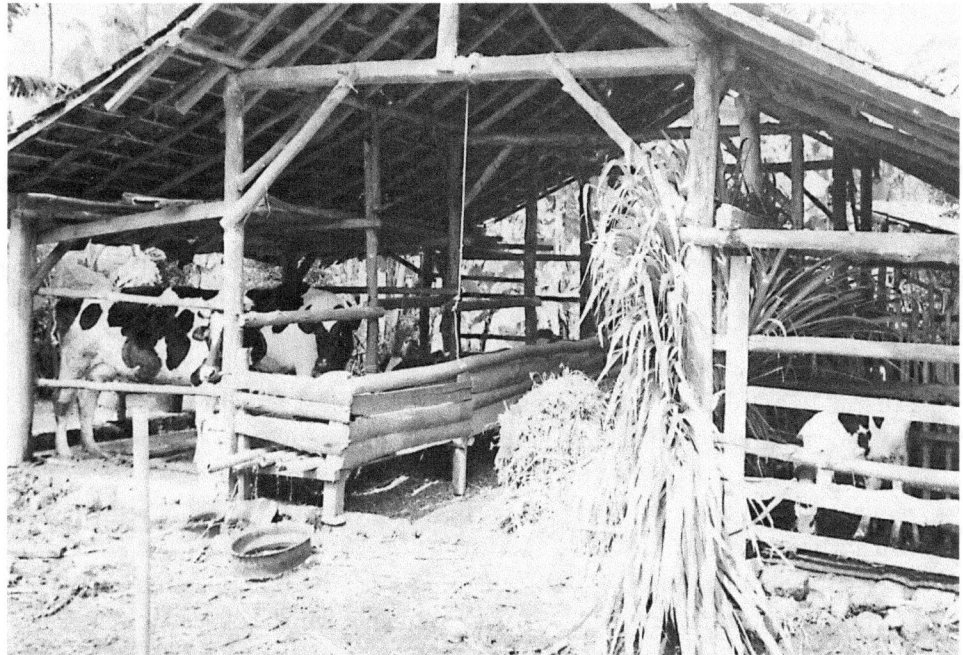

Figure 7.1: A traditional small holder dairy shed in Indonesia.

Asia, purely for the convenience of the farmer whereas free stalls are the most common in more developed dairy industries, because cow comfort is given a higher priority. Although they are usually associated with very large farms, free stall sheds can be designed for herds of any size as described later in this chapter. There are two basic types of housing systems, tie-up housing (tie stalls) and loose housing, which can either be with or without access to free stalls.

7.2.1 Tie stalls

With tie stall systems, each cow is restrained in a separate stall. Feed is delivered in a trough in front of the cows. Milking usually takes place individually in the stall, by hand or machine, the latter using either a bucket or a pipeline system. Manure is collected in a gutter behind the animal. With cows tied up all year round, they can suffer from foot problems and become stiff. Therefore, they should be provided with an easy to clean, soft surface on which to lie down, such as rubber mats or straw. Heat detection demands more attention in tie stalls and a high incidence of trampled teats can become another problem.

As far as the cow is concerned, tie stalls:

- are extremely uncomfortable and often have a hard surface.
- cause pain, with risk of inflammation of knees and hocks.

- are frustrating, because lying down with the head constrained is more difficult and the animal cannot lie down with a stretched foreleg or with its head tucked into its front legs.
- are boring, because they restrict any opportunity for social contact or interaction and foraging.
- restrict the ability for each cow to self-groom, particularly if the tether rope or chain is too short.
- reduce lying and resting time, which can lead to increased lameness.
- can lead to abnormal behaviour, such as swinging from side to side and shifting/moving back and forth. Many cows often stand in a dull state if not eating or otherwise stimulated.
- can lead to more frequent occurrences of stereotypical activities, such as bar biting or tongue rolling, which disappear when animals are transferred to loose housing.
- remove the ability for stock to find the best location in the shed for reducing climatic stresses.
- reduce the quality of the microclimate (higher relative humidity and air ammonia concentration and lower air movement), which can lead to reduced cow comfort and performance (Keidane 2007). As an example, one study (Kate Blaszac, personal communication) reported relative humidities of 94% in tie stalls compared to 74 to 84% in free stalls.
- are all too commonly associated with poor hygiene, meaning that the cow is forced to lie in her own manure, thus creating additional problems with animal health and milking hygiene, such as mastitis.
- can adversely affect reproductive performance, partly because cows cannot move freely and assist in identifying other cows on heat.
- can lead to higher teat injuries due to physical damage.
- can have dimensions that may influence cow behaviour, cleanliness and wellbeing.

If circumstances require that the animal is temporarily tethered, she should be tied with a halter and released as soon as possible. Nasal tying, that is threading a rope through a hole in the nasal septum, can cause irritation and infection. A temporarily tied or single housed animal must always be able to keep at least visual contact with her herd mates to lessen stress reactions. A mirror may even substitute for other cows, for a short time. Some behavioural scientists argue that cows in tie stalls are considered to have had regular exercise if they are released for just one hour per day for two days per week. But one could likewise argue that 'the more exercise the better'. The scoring system we have developed for cow welfare, described in Chapter 8 and Appendix 5, only provides points for good cow welfare if cows are allowed to move freely at least once each day.

If farmers persist with tie stalls, they need to pay closer attention to stall dimensions. Zurbrigg *et al.* (2005) noted that:

- shorter stalls are associated with more cows with dirty hind limbs and rotated hind claws. This is very apparent from several pictures in this book.
- low tie rails can lead to more cows with neck lesions and broken tails, the latter resulting either from the tail being stepped on or forceful manipulation by the farmer.
- short tie ropes or chains can lead to more swollen hocks and dirty hind limbs with cows struggling to stand and lie down easily.

In summary, tie stalls are *not* appropriate for the optimum wellbeing of milking cows and these conditions can negatively affect milk yields and cow longevity. Tie stalls have been the traditional method of maintaining dairy cows in some European countries for many decades. This has created so much public concern that certain countries, such as Norway, have recently legislated against their future use in preference to loose housing.

7.2.2 Loose housing

With loose housing, cows are not tied up and can walk around freely. Such systems usually have a loafing area and a lying area, with the feeding area separated from the lying area. As the cows are forced to walk frequently, the manure is spread over a large floor area so has to be collected by scraping the dung by hand (or sometimes mechanically) into a manure pit. With adequate water supplies, rapid flushing of large amounts of water can clean alleys, directing effluent into a pond. Milking is usually carried out in a specific milking parlour or area in the shed. The feed trough is separated from the loafing alley by either a feeding rack or wire rope.

Loose housing can be of two types, either with a common lying area with open lounging or with cubicles or free stalls.

- In open lounging systems, cows can lie down anywhere, although they are usually allocated a particular place to rest. The floor can be earthen or cement, generally with bedding material, the base being well drained. In dry climates, earthen floors without bedding can be used so long as the dry manure is frequently removed. The loafing area behind the feed troughs should be cement and at least 3 m wide. Each cow should be allocated at least 9 m^2 resting area.
- Open lounges create their own problems of regularly removing and cleaning the bedding and ensuring all cows will use it in preference to lying on dirty cement walkways, which increases the potential for mastitis problems.
- 'Compost barns' are becoming popular in which the fresh manure is removed at least daily and the dried manure is regularly turned over to create a type of compost bedding which remains dry and relatively free of pathogens.

7.2.3   Free stalls

A free stall shed is essentially a feedpad with the addition of specific bedding areas where the stock can lie down. It is generally a covered shed and may include a loafing area for cattle to also be loose housed where they can stand, ruminate or idle. In these sheds each cow is provided with a stall that she may enter and leave at will.

When well designed and managed, free stalls provide the ideal system for intensively managing dairy cows off pasture as each animal is provided with a specific place to rest, their management (feeding, cleaning and relaxing) is potentially optimised and the system can operate efficiently with minimal labour. However, they are relatively expensive to construct and can become very unprofitable if cows suffer from poor welfare, animal health issues and reduced milk quality due to poor feeding and herd management. If there is at least one comfortable stall available per cow, weaker and low status cows will have fewer problems with feed intake, water intake and lameness.

Stalls must allow enough room for the largest cow to freely enter the stall, lie down, rest comfortably and easily get to her feet to exit the stall. To do this, stalls should take into account the cow's normal desire to rest facing uphill slightly and change resting positions or stretch while lying down. In addition, there needs to be sufficient room at the front of the stall as cows need to lunge forward to lift their hindquarters first when rising.

Free stalls should be seen as individual cow bedding cubicles where partitions orientate stock for comfort and sanitation, providing each cow with a dry and comfortable place to lie down and rest and ruminate. Free stall sheds should have one stall for each lactating cow. Some farmers provide additional stalls to allow for herd growth and to provide areas for subordinate animals to move away from more aggressive herd mates.

Stalls can be arranged in a single row or in more than one row with a central feeding alley or with feeding alleys along the sidewalls. They can be arranged with cows facing one another (head-to-head) or the other way around (tail-to-tail). With the tail-to-tail arrangement, a central cow alley, 2.2 m wide between the cubicles is needed. If the stalls are head-to-head, two cow alleys behind each row are necessary. Usually one of these alleys is combined with the feed alley. Free stalls are usually laid out in modules with crossovers providing access to the feeding alley. These can provide multiple routes between cubicles and feeding area and so minimise the adverse effects that dominant stock can have on the eating behaviour of submissive stock.

Stall dimensions should be based on the largest 25% of the herd to allow for increase in cow size through improved feeding and genetics over time. They should also provide for adequate lying down as well as necessary forward and sideways lunging to stand. Typical Friesians require about 240 cm long × 120 cm wide lying space with a further 60 cm forward lunging to allow for normal standing behaviour. Forward lunging space can be shared where two rows of stalls face head to head.

The size of the cubicles depends on cow size. For cows:

- weighing 400–500 kg, they should be 104–109 cm wide and 198–208 cm long
- weighing 500–590 kg, they should be 109–114 cm wide and 208–218 cm long
- weighing 590–680 kg, they should be 114–122 cm wide and 229–244 cm long.

Stalls that are too long or wide allow the animal to move forward, in which case faeces and urine can be deposited within the stall and not in the alleyway. To further prevent cows from soiling the cubicles, shoulder and neck rails are needed to force cows backwards when they stand up. The distance of the adjustable shoulder rail to the back of the cubicle, measured diagonally, should be about 1.8 m, and the height to the cubicle floor may vary between 0.9 and 1.05 m. Cow trainers, electric wires above the stalls are sometimes installed to train cows not to soil their stalls.

The stall curb separates the stall area from manure in the walkway. It should be high enough to prevent manure from entering the stalls, but low enough to allow cows to enter and exit the stalls easily. Recommended maximum curb heights are 20 cm or, if a mattress or mat is used, 30 cm.

The condition of the bedding is most important to encourage cows to use the stalls. The free stall base and bedding should provide a comfortable conforming surface to cushion the cow as she drops to a resting position or while resting (Graves *et al.* 2009). When cows are forced to lie on hard surfaces, they do not lie down for long, are more unsettled and may develop knee and hock lesions and swelling. All base types need loose bedding material on top for further cushioning, moisture absorption and to reduce friction. If the stall base provides good cushioning, less bedding is needed on top. To be comfortable, the base and bedding layers should cushion the contact areas for hock, knees, hips, brisket and shoulders. It is best to provide cushioning using a thick layer (15 to 20 cm) of bedding on a firm base or by an intermediate layer, cushioning mat or mattress and 3 to 5 cm of bedding. Ideally, if only using a rubber mattress, it should be 5 cm thick for optimum comfort. Rubber mats are common and can vary in thickness for < 10 mm to > 25 mm. The thicker the rubber mat, the greater its degree of flexibility (and presumably comfort) for the cow when she lies down. Mattresses are made by putting a resilient fill material such as crumb rubber, foam or liquid inside a woven polyethylene or felt-type geotextile textile material.

Hard rubber mats provide little cushioning, particularly if very thin, and they may be slippery. Soft rubber mats provide the same features as mattresses. Attachment methods, surface texture and compaction of the mat or mattress material are all issues to consider when selecting and installing mats or mattresses. Bedding is required on top of mattresses and mats to help to maintain clean dry conditions.

In addition to preventing injury and providing comfort for cows, free stall bases should only require minimum maintenance. Materials used for bases vary from stone-free earth fill, available on site, to sand, to concrete. Earth fill requires the most maintenance as cows getting up and down will disturb and hollow out the surface. It is essential to select a material that does not contain stones or other solid particles that can be kicked into walkways, potentially causing injury or discomfort to cows' hooves.

Sand is the most favoured bedding as it reduces pressure on the joints, distributes weight over the area and provides unparalleled traction. It must not be too fine and should be free of rocks and pebbles. Sand-filled stalls need to be kept full to encourage their maximum usage. Sand is easily pushed around by cows, it has a high labour requirement for manure handling and can quickly contaminate walkways and so fill up manure storage tanks. Being very abrasive, it can damage manure pumps, so it should not be used with mechanical or liquid manure handling systems. Although hard surfaces such as concrete and hard rubber mats do not hollow out, they are less comfortable and so reduce lying times, can increase the chance of injuries (such as lameness, hock damage and pressure sores), and will lead to stall refusal.

Common base materials include:

- hard packed earth
- sand
- concrete
- mattresses
- hard and soft rubber mats.

Regardless of base material, a layer of bedding material is needed. This provides additional cushioning, absorbs moisture, helps keep cows clean and restricts bacterial growth. Low cost and ease of handling are desirable. Mixtures of different bedding materials should also be considered. Various organic and inorganic materials are used for bedding such as:

- organic: rice hulls, sawdust, straw, hay, wood shavings, cornstalks, peanut hulls, chopped or shredded paper, recycled manure solids
- inorganic: sand, limestone screenings, field lime, gypsum
- waterbeds seem to be the most preferred bedding in temperate winters, probably because of their warmth when artificially heated.

Manure and wet bedding should be removed and replaced with dry bedding material each day. Cleaning should be frequent enough to keep the back of the stall clean because this is where the cow's udder and teats are in contact with the bedding when she lies down. Organic bedding should be added every 1–3 days, especially on mattresses and rubber mats, as it is hard to keep bedding on these surfaces.

Dirty cow alleys will result in dirty beds and udders, weakened hoof horn and potential mastitis. Cow and feed alleys should be kept clean by manual scraping, automatic scrapers or flood washing. Although cows can still be in their stalls, it is better to time flood washing during milking when they are away from the shed.

Care should be taken to ensure the stall construction or installation does not interfere with either the natural movements of the rising and reclining cows or the ventilation of the shed. Consider the effects of the stall structure on air flow at cow level. For example, using smaller dimensional steel rather than larger wooden planks when constructing the stalls, can result in a more open area for better ventilation.

The free stall environment should be made safe for the stock through ensuring they cannot put their heads through gates and fences or get stuck under stall divisions and barriers. There should be no projections, such as broken boards or rails or rough, sharp edges on the concrete. Rails should be strong enough not to break when cows lean on them. Walking surfaces can be grooved to minimise slips and falls and so encourage normal oestrus activity.

The free stall facility should be designed to ensure smooth and quiet cow flow. There should be no sudden changes from light to dark, reflections or drains across the cow alleys. Cows will move more smoothly along curved races, up a slight incline and where they have 'sure' footing. Gates could be muffled by attaching rubber strips to prevent excessive noise. Yards must be designed for easy drafting of targeted cows as this activity causes stress. Stock should only be moved around using 'flappers' (leather strips attached to a cane, sometimes known as cattle talkers) rather than using wooden or metal pickets or pipes. Excessive twisting of an animal's tail is unacceptable and electric prods should only be used in emergencies.

Proper selection of stall dimensions, partition, design, stall base type and bedding material is essential in encouraging their daily use but regular management and maintenance are necessary to assure clean, comfortable cows. Check stalls at least three times daily (at milking and feeding), remove manure and wet material and rearrange bedding, if necessary, to provide a uniform surface. Adding large amounts of bedding material less frequently is not economical. It can lead to increased bedding waste – the material can be soiled or wet soon after spreading in the stall which can reduce cow comfort and lead to undesirable cow positioning before the next bedding application.

As organic bedding can more readily support bacterial contamination than can inorganic material, it should be replaced more frequently, with soiled organic material removed from the rear third of the stall every day. The first step a cow takes into the stall is the place the udder and teats will rest as she settles down into her lying position. The regular cleaning of walkways can reduce manure tracked into the stall. Depending on the frequency of milking and on the movement of the cows, cleaning the walkways up to three times a day can be appropriate.

7.2.4　Monitoring free stall use

The cow is the final inspector of free stalls and if cows are not successfully and regularly using them, or they are dirty and show signs of injury, action is required. There are a variety of ways to monitor the cows' use of free stalls and free stall sheds, such as:

- Do cows appear comfortable when standing or lying? If not, stall dimensions and bedding may need attention.
- Do cows have to push, bang and/or bump against stall components to lie down, get up or change positions?
- Do cows lie backwards in the stalls or in the alleys?
- Do cows stand half-in or half-out of the stalls? This can occur when the stalls are too short, the neck rail is too far back or when the stalls are otherwise uncomfortable.
- Do cows stand in the stalls in an angular fashion? This indicates the stalls are too wide.
- Are all stalls used equally? If not, there would be a reason why some are not chosen by the cows.
- When cows normally rest (between 10 p.m. and 4 a.m.) are more than 20 to 30% of the herd standing in the stalls? If so, stall comfort may be questionable.
- Are cows' udders, tails or hindquarters dirty? This could indicate dirty bedding but may also be due to low fibre diets and very loose manure.
- Are there patches of rubbed off hair or visible injuries to hocks and knees? These are signs that cows rub excessively on stall partitions or neck rails when rising or lying down.
- Are cows walking very slowly, or timidly, with rear feet spread wide? This could be a sign of poor traction or laminitis.
- Are some cows slipping and falling in the shed? This could also be a sign of poor traction.
- The comfort of the stall bedding can be assessed by the
  - ➤ Wet knee test, which involves kneeling in the stall for 10 s and if the knee is wet, the stall bedding is not dry enough.
  - ➤ Drop knee test, which involves crouching and then dropping to your knees in the stall. Any pain reaction in your knees will quickly tell you how truly comfortable the stalls are.

- Do more than 20% of the cows defecate in the milking parlour? This could indicate discomfort or uneasiness in the free stall shed.
- Are cows bellowing excessively or exhibiting abnormal behaviour? This also requires attention as discussed in Chapter 4.

7.2.5   Straw yards

A straw yard offers cows a very comfortable bed provided the yard is well managed and used properly. This means no overcrowding and making sure the bed is firm and dry. The quality of the straw yard depends on:

- Straw management: the bed should support the cow's weight as she walks. Absorbent, clean and dry straw should be added at least once each day and mouldy or dusty straw should be avoided.
- Fluids: how much is added with urine, dung, water spillages and rain and how much is removed as slurry, evaporation and other ways?
- Stocking density and cattle movement: how often do cows stand and walk in particular areas as busy areas get wet?
- At least once each day add 1 kg straw/m^2 and double this amount after cleaning out the yard. Another way of calculating is 1 m^2 of bedded straw per 1000 L annual milk production with 6 kg per cow per day as the minimum.
- Straw yards can be monitored by assessing how dirty the cows are or by counting the number of udder wipes needed during milking.
- The amount of dirt (dung) on the cow gives an idea of the level of hygiene in the straw yards.

7.3   Other cowshed equipment

7.3.1   Cow cooling equipment

This has been discussed fully in other books written by the senior author, as in Chapter 19 of Moran (2005) and Chapter 12 of Moran (2012a).

7.3.2   Facilities and equipment for young stock

These have been described in detail in Chapter 7 of Moran (2012b).

7.3.3   Facilities and equipment for additional health care

To ensure good health care, sufficient health facilities are needed and cowsheds should include additional stalls for such purposes. These and other stock handling aids are included in the following list:

- Treatment area, for confining animals on heat, artificial insemination, routine health checks, pregnancy diagnosis and examining sick cows. As animals are usually separated when they leave the milking parlour, it should be located close to it. The width of this treatment area should be at least 0.7 m per cow and the length 3 m. It is convenient to store equipment in a specific veterinary drug box in this treatment area for treating hoof problems, for trimming hoofs, taking blood samples etc. There should be one treatment stall for every 20 cow stalls (with a minimum of two stalls).

- Separation area or hospital pens, to treat sick cows properly and prevent the spread of disease. It should be located close to the milking parlour. Drinking water should be available, with concrete floor and gutters to allow for frequent cleaning and sanitising. Ideally it should also have a shelf above ground level for storing medicines and other cow health-related equipment. There should be one treatment stall per 30 stalls (with a minimum of two stalls). With tie stalls, there is little need for a special separation area.
- Calving area, to permit proper attention at this critical time. With loose housing, cows may need to be tied up in stalls and should calve down away from the milking herd and close by the calf pens. As with the separation area, ease and thoroughness of cleaning and sanitation are key features. There should be one calving stall per 30 stalls (with a minimum of two stalls).
- Separate bull and mating pen. If using natural mating, bulls must be isolated from other stock except when mating. In fully stocked cowsheds, it may be preferable to bring the cow on heat, once identified, to the bull and so provide room for mating activities in the bull pen rather than let the bull mate in the laneway or a free stall.
- Cattle race, crush and/or head bales or other ways of immobilising stock are important both for the stock (to reduce stress) and the staff (to reduce injury). A cattle race allows stock to be separated out and immobilised when requiring additional attention such as insemination, veterinary treatment or foot trimming. Cattle crushes and head gates should be well designed to ensure that stock can be examined without fear of injury. Head bales should be made of pipes with sufficient robustness to hold a large unsettled animal.
- Footbaths should be available for routine hoof treatment, at least 2 to 3 m in length and 0.15 m deep. The width should be the same as the passage to prevent cows from bypassing the bath without using it. Double footbaths are better because they allow dirt to be washed off before treatment. The first bath tends to activate the dunging reflex which allows the solution in the second foot bath to stay effective for longer. A solid platform of 3 m between footbaths will help get rid of some of the wash solution from the first footbath. Emptying and refilling them should be quick and easy. Hulsen (2013) recommends that footbaths should contain 4% formalin or 38% commercial formaldehyde solution. Each cow should walk through them once each week. The frequency should vary depending on hoof cleanliness and dryness and how much they show evidence of horn erosion or digital dermatitis.

- Electric cow trainers. These consist of wires positioned above stalls that carry electricity and are used to teach cows to step backwards when their back is arched before defecation and urination. They then alter behaviour and keep cows and stalls cleaner. They are, however, risk factors for silent heats, clinical mastitis, ketosis and culling, with herds not using cow trainers having fewer of these issues. In some poorly designed stalls, cows prefer to stand and so do not have to experience the pain associated with lying and rising. When they are moved to better designed stalls, the cows use the trainers.

7.3.4 High cost equipment

This book is primarily about small holder dairy (SHD) farmers but this section covers some larger-scale investments in improving cow comfort on bigger farms. Such items will improve cow comfort and can become important factors beneficially influencing herd contentment in large sheds where there is likely to be increased competition between cows. There are considerably more antagonistic interactions within a herd of several hundred dairy cows than within a 5 or 10 cow dairy herd, so having this sort of equipment can reduce negative interactions.

- *Rotating cow brushes* are sometimes provided to allow cows to groom and scratch themselves. It may also reduce frustration or stress due to boredom. Cows can be very vigorous in their use of brushes so they need to be quite robust. Generally cows need little behavioural enrichment because feeding, ruminating and resting occupy most of their time and they can rely on other cows for social stimulation. Some of the brushes automatically start rotating when an approaching cow is detected. Generally cows use brushes to scratch their backs rather than their heads so they should be positioned at the right height.
- *Self-locking gates* are designed to restrain cows as they put their head down to eat from the feed bunk. Some free stall sheds have self-catching lockable feeding head-stalls along the feed line to allow animals to be caught for veterinary attention, insemination or even locked away from the feed.
  These confine the cow in order to facilitate closer observation or individual management. In addition, they reduce aggressive interactions and displacement of socially subordinate cows while eating. When they have an option, cows do not choose these self-locking gates. Despite this, when forced to use them, they have little impact on daily feed intakes, milk yields, levels of mastitis and signs of stress.
- *Cow showers* can be designed to be activated either manually or automatically. In the latter, the showering and interval cycles are triggered only when the dual motion sensors detect an animal is present and the air temperature is above a specified threshold. As air temperatures increase, the interval time

automatically decreases, thus giving animals more frequent shower cycles to reduce heat stress. By using a high capacity, coarse droplet shower nozzle, enough water can be applied to fully wet the cows to the hide. Mist and fogging nozzles work by cooling the air around the cows and the disadvantage is that the mist can be easily blown away under windy conditions, or when used with fans. If a mist or fog builds up on the cow's hair coat, it can also trap a layer of air between the skin and the water, which holds in body heat. In comparison, soaker nozzles produce a coarse droplet spray, which penetrates the hair and wets the cow's hide.

There should be a continuous flow of air over the backs of the cattle any time the cooling system is in operation. This causes the water to evaporate, which takes the heat away from the cattle in the process. Fans can be controlled separately from the cooling system, and are set to operate continuously above a temperature of 21°C.

Normal recommendations are to shower the animals for a short period of time, 0.5 to 3 min, to soak the hide. After the shower shuts off, fans evaporate the water off the cattle by blowing across their backs for 5 to 15 min, before repeating the shower cycle. Common locations for installing a shower cooling system are in the holding pen area, where cows are crowded together tightly, and in the feed line area, but not so it will spray into the feed line or a stall.

7.4   Examples of complete cow housing systems

Many SHD farm systems and cowsheds are not purpose built but evolve over time, often without adequate long-term planning. They are frequently constructed out of the cheapest materials available and, all too often, without consideration of the long-term ramifications of using such poor quality materials. Additional inputs include the need to eventually purchase better quality materials and the time and labour required to renovate poorly constructed sheds. Therefore, careful planning and discussions with other farmers and service providers are time well spent when constructing or renovating a cowshed. When visiting other farmers, one good question to ask is *What would you have done differently, with hindsight, now that your shed is up and running?* The reader is directed to the following chapter (Section 8.2.2) that reports the recent study of Nguhiu-Mwangi *et al.* (2013). They found that poor cow welfare could be directly attributed to poor planning and construction of sheds on SHD farms in Nairobi, Kenya.

The following are plans and pictures of well designed and constructed SHD sheds. Many small holder farmers start with one or two cows and become 'part-time' dairy farmers depending on other off-farm or farming enterprises to provide additional income streams. In SE Asia, it is generally considered that to become a full-time dairy farmer in which incomes originate completely from the dairy enterprise, farmers require 8 to 10 milking cows, plus the necessary replacement stock. Therefore, it seems logical to construct a cowshed to house such a number of milking cows and young stock. If the resources do not allow for its construction at the one time, at least space should be left for expansion at a later date.

Loose housing with free stalls and an outside exercise yard for night-time resting would provide the basics of a well managed and 'cow friendly' system. The following examples are of eight cow (Sri Lanka) and six cow (Vietnam) free stall sheds but their slightly modified construction could increase their capacity to house 10 or more milking cows.

7.4.1 Sri Lankan example

Figure 7.2 presents the plans for an eight milking cow free stall shed with a separate milking parlour and calf and heifer facilities. There is also an outside sand yard for night-time resting. This plan was developed by our colleague Jim Burrell.

The dairy design is flexible and able to be extended through the body of the dairy as the numbers of milking cows expand. Dry cows and adult heifers can be accommodated in another simple shed as an annexe to the sand yard if needed.

7.4.2 Vietnam example

Figures 7.3a–e are of a durable six cow free stall shed in Vietnam while Figure 7.3f is of an associated calf and heifer shed. Considerable use has been made from local materials. The uprights, roof beams and two of the free stalls are made from treated wood, although they may not be longlasting in regions severely infested with white ants, while the roof is made from local palm fronds. Each day, the manure can be easily cleaned from the outside sand yard.

More conventional longlasting materials used include rubber mats for the free stalls, concrete for the floor and water trough, and pipes for the feeding gates and some of the free stalls. Figure 7.3f of the calf and heifer shed includes a small horizontal feed mixer into which machine-chopped grass is incorporated with concentrates to produce a total mixed ration for all the stock. Depending on its location, cow comfort in this shed would benefit from the installation of fans, and even a sprinkler system.

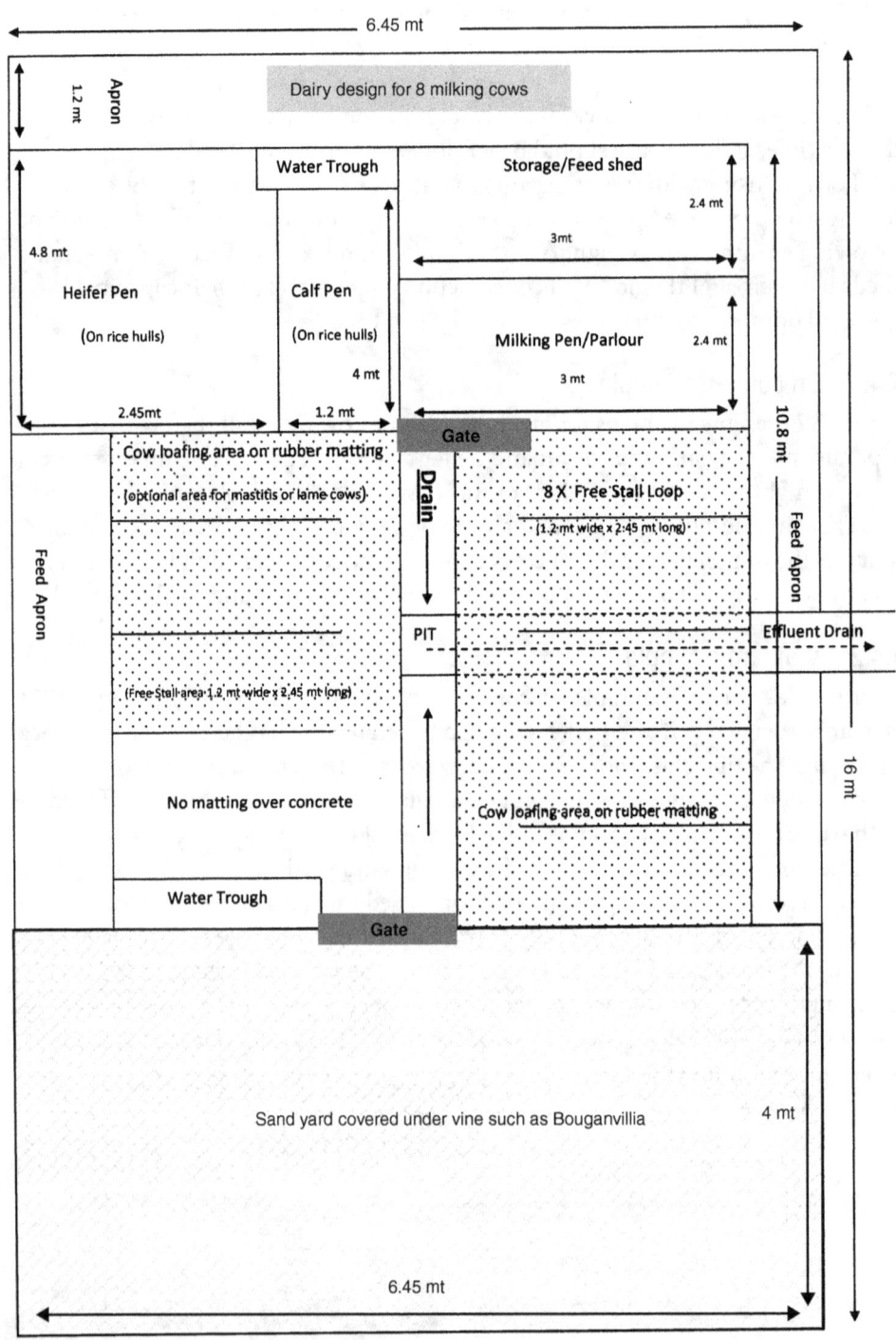

Figure 7.2: Floor plans for an eight cow free stall.

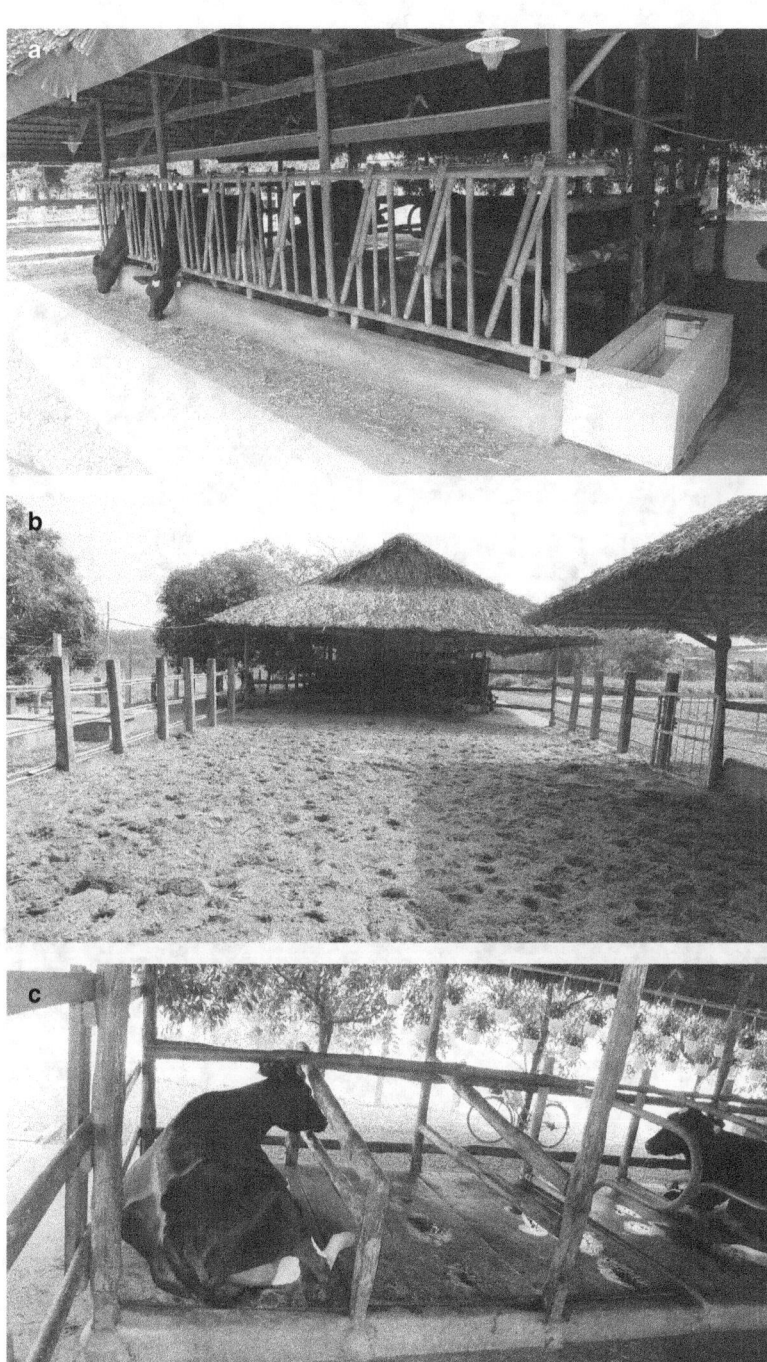

Figure 7.3: A six cow free stall shed in Vietnam. a) The feeding face. b) The outdoor sand yard for night-time resting. c) A cow lying in one of the free stalls. d) Inside the shed. e) Inside the shed. f) Associated calf and heifer shed.

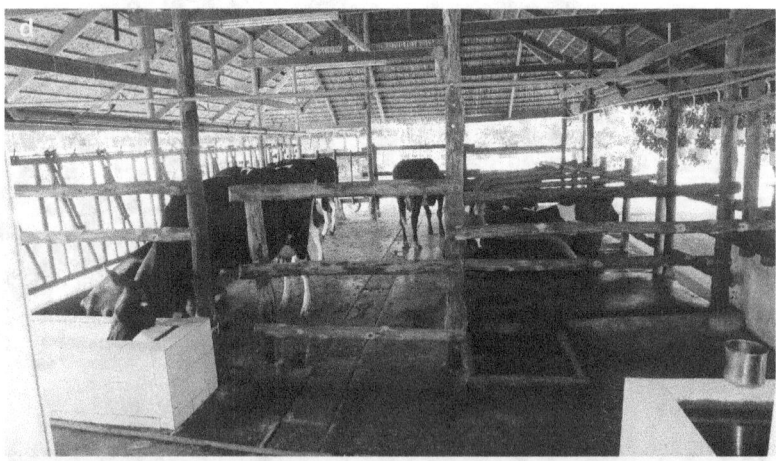

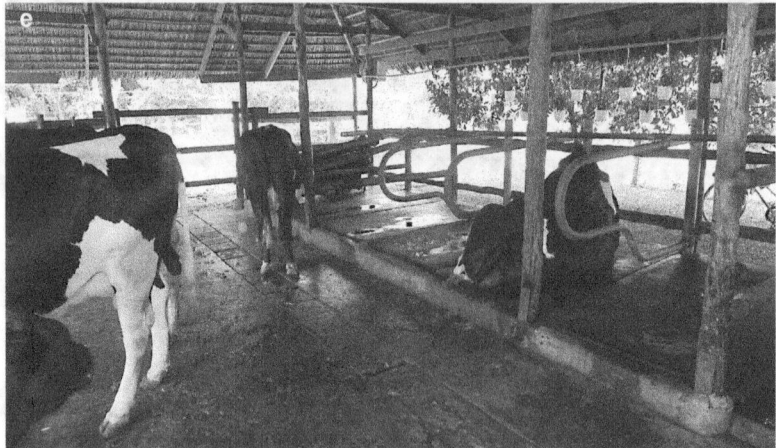

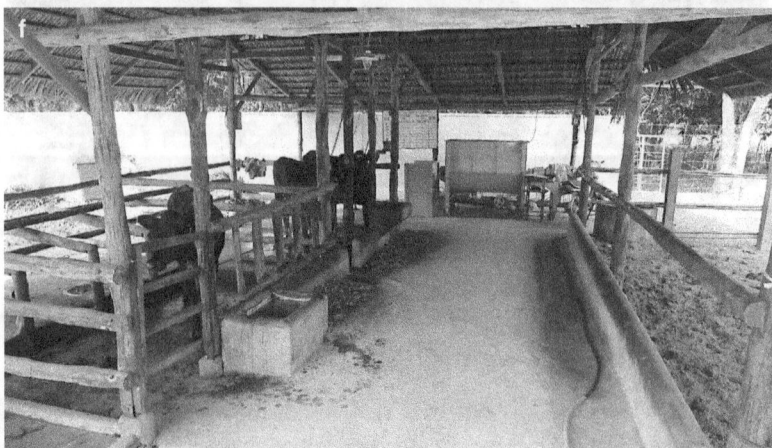

Figure 7.3: Continued

8

Auditing cow welfare

This chapter presents a series of frameworks to help assess the state of a cow's welfare.

The main points of this chapter

- The five basic freedoms for good animal welfare are freedom from hunger and thirst, discomfort, pain, fear and distress as well as the freedom to express normal behaviour. These form the basic elements of many animal welfare protocols.
- Direct animal measurements are good indicators of an animal's current wellbeing and help identify longer-term animal welfare problems. These should integrate long-term consequences of past husbandry practices, be non-intrusive, and free from observer bias.
- A generic welfare assessment protocol is presented and can be used to evaluate the welfare practices on small holder dairy (SHD) farms.
- This chapter also presents two case studies. The first, evaluating animal welfare at 53 large-scale dairy farms in the UK, clearly demonstrates the enormous ranges in quantifiable cow welfare indicators, highlighting lameness to be a significant issue on most farms. It also shows that

while some farms were obviously worse than others, overall there were no thoroughly 'good' or 'bad' farms.
- The second case study, which investigates 112 SHD farms in Kenya, attributes many of the observed cow welfare problems to poor housing design and farmer ignorance.
- The second study also highlighted the farmers' very poor perception of cow welfare with most believing that animal suffering and its alleviation was not important and that animal comfort was unnecessary.

Traditionally, farm animal welfare audits have focused on the measurements of resources provided to the animal such as housing-related facilities, management practices and human–animal relationships. These are often difficult to quantify and may not necessarily result in improved standards of animal welfare although they can indicate risks or reasons for the animal's welfare. More direct animal measurements, such as behaviour and health, can be taken as better indicators of their current wellbeing and help identify longer-term animal welfare problems.

8.1   Indicators of animal welfare

Many different methods can be used to measure an animal's welfare, and a balance needs to be sought so that enough measures are taken to be rigorous, that the measures are scientifically based and that the data can be collected in a timely manner. When choosing direct measures of welfare, several factors need to be considered. Indicators should integrate the long-term consequences of past husbandry practices. They should be non-intrusive, so as to cause minimal disturbance to the animal's natural behaviour. They must be reasonably free of observer bias. They should highlight welfare problems and identify failures in farm management that contributed to such problems.

Welfare observations should then be centred around three aspects:

- Validity. *What does this indicator tell us about the animal's welfare state?*
- Repeatability. *Do different observers always see the same problem?*
- Feasibility. *How easy is it to record this indicator?*

Most approaches to welfare assessment are based on indicators of reduced welfare. Understandably this is because the greatest compromise to welfare lies with negative situations. However, it is also worthwhile putting more emphasis on indicators of *good* welfare. Farmers providing a non-stressful environment for the cows to live in and positive social interactions would be considered the main components of good welfare. Social and non-social play in calves or social licking in adult cows are examples of positive social activities, and stock are only motivated to perform such behaviours once the animal's primary needs are satisfied. Animal welfare research and assessment are moving in this direction, and more objective indicators of positive welfare will be developed with time.

8.1.1 Five basic freedoms of livestock

The welfare requirements of cattle can best be summarised in the 'five freedoms' (Farm Animal Welfare Council 2009). These were originally developed by the UK government as a part of a report into farm animal welfare (Brambell 1965) but are now applied to all animals under the care of humans. These five freedoms are as follows:

1. Freedom from hunger and thirst, through ready access to fresh water and a diet to maintain full health and vigour.
2. Freedom from discomfort, through provision of appropriate shelter and comfortable resting areas.
3. Freedom from pain, by prevention and, when sick, rapid diagnosis and treatment.
4. Freedom from fear and distress by ensuring the animal lives in conditions that avoid mental suffering.
5. Freedom to express normal behaviour by providing adequate space, proper facilities and the company of other animals.

These five freedoms address both physical fitness and mental suffering and are best viewed as a practical, comprehensive checklist to assess the strengths and weaknesses of any husbandry system. There is a hierarchy of needs in cattle and the five freedoms should not be taken to imply that all animals should be free from exposure to any stress, ever. The aim is not to eliminate stress but to prevent suffering and to progress towards improved welfare by providing for the animal's needs. Suffering occurs when animals fail or have difficulty in coping with stress. All dairy cattle management and housing systems should be designed, constructed, maintained and managed to assist with these 'five freedoms'. In addition, they provide the framework of the recommended protocol for welfare of dairy stock on tropical SHD farms detailed in Chapter 10 of this manual.

8.1.2 Key Performance Indicators of cattle welfare

Key Performance Indicators (KPI) can act as a guide to help farmers diagnose the strengths and weaknesses in their dairy enterprise. In simple terms, KPIs are then diagnostic tools to help identify weaknesses adversely affecting farm performance. Farmers can use these indicators to identify areas of animal welfare weaknesses, and help to give them an idea of their performance in relation to other farms.

Comparing between farms can be a useful way to bring about changes, as farmers are more likely to try to improve their management practices if they can identify where they are compared to others in terms of welfare and productivity. There are various KPIs available for SHD farmers that cover health, productivity and welfare, and many of these have been highlighted by Moran (2009b).

The Welfare Quality (2009) project has listed 12 such KPIs that relate to animal welfare. This is specifically for the first four 'basic freedoms of livestock', as the fifth freedom, to express natural behaviour, should be assured if all else is satisfied (see Figures 8.1, 8.2 and 8.3).

1. Animals should not suffer from prolonged hunger.
2. Animals should not suffer from prolonged thirst.
3. Animals should be comfortable, especially within their lying areas.
4. Animals should be in a good thermal environment.
5. Animals should be able to move around freely.
6. Animals should not be physically injured.
7. Animals should be free of disease.

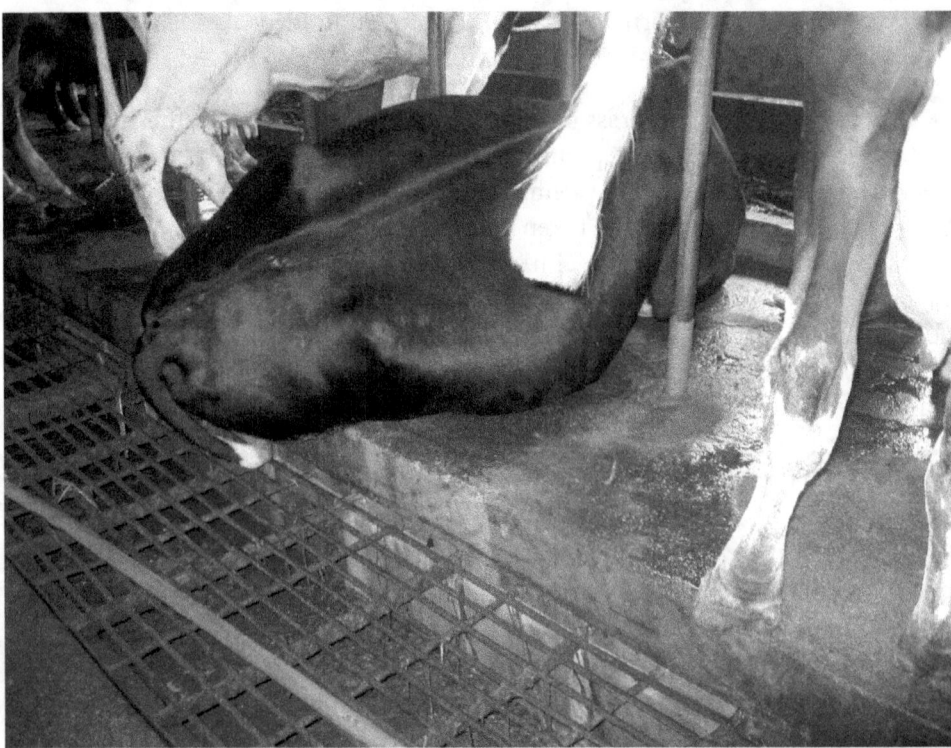

Figure 8.1: These free stalls are too short and have no soft bedding.

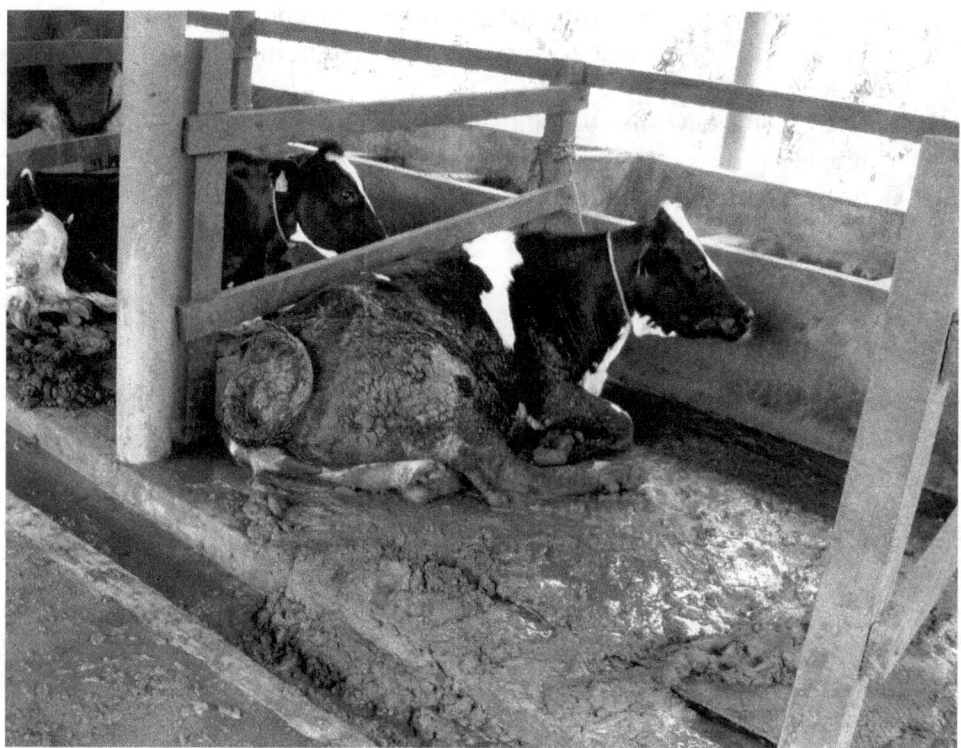

Figure 8.2: These cows are permanently tethered with appalling hygiene.

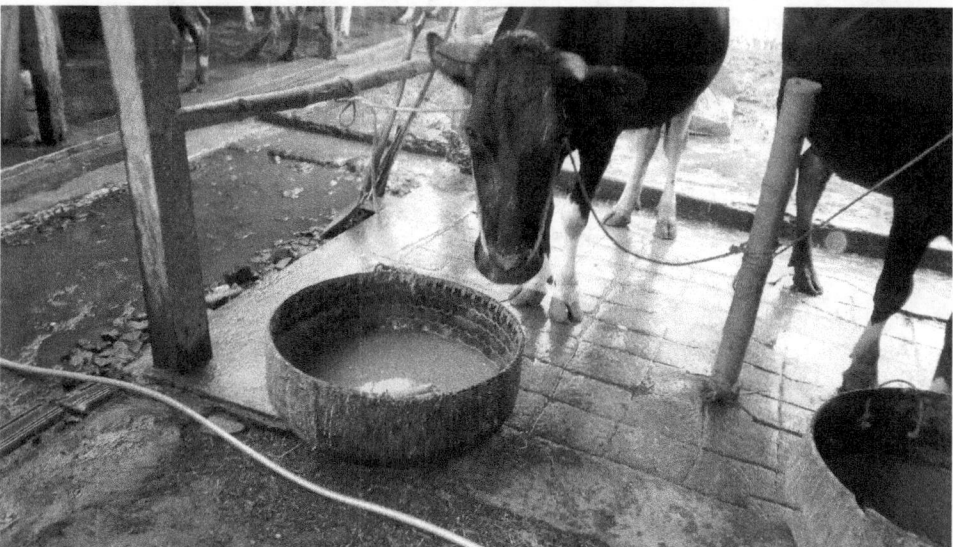

Figure 8.3: A very common problem in many tropical small holder farms, no clean drinking water, only mixed in as a slurry with the concentrates and only offered twice each day.

8. Animals should not suffer from pain induced by inappropriate management.
9. Animals should be allowed to express natural, non-harmful, social behaviours.
10. Animals should have the possibility of expressing other intuitively desirable natural behaviours such as exploration and play.
11. Good human–animal relationships are beneficial to the welfare of animals.
12. Animals should not experience negative emotions such as fear, distress, frustration or apathy.

It is noted that these KPIs are without quantitative descriptors, making it difficult to ensure repeatability of measures if using this list alone. Full details on how these KPIs can be measured are available online, and the reference for this is given in the list of References at the end of this book.

8.1.3   A simplified scoring system for assessing dairy cow welfare

We have developed the key issues highlighted above into a simplified 'farmer friendly' scoring system to assess dairy cow welfare (presented in Table 8.1) that we believe is well suited to the thousands of SHD farmers throughout Asia. It contains 36 questions or observations, is based on the 'five freedoms of animal welfare' and addresses both tethering and loose housing. The questionnaire is a combination of different auditing systems for dairy cattle, including those from World Society for the Protection of Animals (WSPA) (Blaszak 2011), AssureWel (2010), Welfare Quality (2009) and Food and Agriculture Organisation (2011). It has been developed to focus more on good rather than poor animal welfare, so the higher the score, the better the welfare for the animals. Because many SHD farmers have few milking cows, we have used 0%, 30% and 90% of the herd as criteria of good stock welfare practices. Tables 8.1 and 8.2 have also been presented as Appendix 5 for ease of copying for distribution to other dairy stakeholders.

How to use this scoring system
1. Complete the details on farm. Animal numbers are important for score calculations.
2. Each of the 'five basic freedoms of animal welfare' is assessed.
3. Each measure is assigned a total of 1.0. The total for each freedom is scored according to the number of measures answered. If the measure does not apply to that particular farm (for example, it may not have any young calves), this should not be taken into account in the total.
4. For each measure, when 'yes' applies to more than 90% of animals, 1.0 points are scored. When 'yes' applies to 30% or less of animals, 0.0 points are scored. When 'yes' applies to 30–90% of animals, 0.5 points are scored.

Table 8.1. A simplified dairy farm animal welfare assessment form.

Details of farm	
Farm location	
Cooperative or feedlot	
Date and time of visit	
Owner/person responsible	
Total number of milking cows on farm	
Total number of calves on farm	
Measure	**Score**
1. Freedom from hunger and thirst	
Do all animals (including calves) have continuous access to water?	
Are all feeders and drinkers functional?	
Are feeders and drinkers clean?	
Are cows in a body condition score between 2 and 4 out of 5 (Chapter 6.1)?	
Do cows have a rumen score appropriate to their point of calving (Chapter 6.6)?	
Are calves fed colostrum?	
Are cows fed a quality mixed ration?	
TOTAL	
2. Freedom from discomfort	
Do cows have a cleanliness score of 2 or less out of 5 (Chapter 6.5)?	
Is bedding provided?	
Is bedding clean and deep enough for cows to lie comfortably?	
Can animals lie down and get up easily?	
Is there shelter from extreme weather?	
Are cows free from hock sores?	
Are cows free from pressure sores?	
Are cows free from any signs of heat stress (< 70 breaths per minute)?	
TOTAL	
3. Freedom from pain, injury and disease	
Are cows free from injuries on their bodies?	
Do cows have a locomotion score of 2 or less out of 5 (Chapter 6.2)?	
Are cows free from clinical disease?	
Do cows have healthy hooves (e.g. no incidences of the diseases described in Chapter 6.3)?	
Do cows have clean, healthy-looking udders?	
Do cows have teat scores of 2 or less out of 4 (Chapter 6.8)?	
Do cows have their tails intact?	
Have calves been disbudded (not dehorned)?	
Have male calves been castrated at 3 months of age or less?	
TOTAL	

(Continued)

Table 8.1. Continued

4. Freedom from fear and distress	
Do cows approach the stockperson?	
Do calves approach the stockperson?	
Will the cows let the stockperson approach within 3 m?	
Can cows be moved gently, without hitting, yelling?	
Will cows walk slowly, not run, when encouraged to move by the stockperson?	
TOTAL	
5. Freedom to express normal behaviour	
Are cows free to move (untethered)?	
If tethered, are cows given access to move freely each day?	
Are calves housed in appropriate groups (between 2 and 8)?	
Can animals turn around fully in their cubicle?	
Is there a minimum of dry lying area of 3.5 m² for adult cattle/bulls and 2.5 m² for growing heifers?	
Is there evidence of normal social behaviours (limited aggressive interactions during feeding and resting)?	
Are stereotypical behaviours minimal?	
TOTAL	

5. Methods for scoring body condition, rumen fill, cleanliness, locomotion, hooves and teat scores are provided in Chapter 6.

6. Appendix 5 presents a second copy of the scoring system for copying and use on farm.

Once this form was developed, the next step was to make a value judgement as to the quality of animal welfare on that particular farm. This step is still evolving because we first need to collect sufficient on-farm data to quantify the range of farm assessment scores likely to be encountered; this may lead to some modifications and improvements in the type of data collected. Not every question can be answered for every farm, so it is not possible to develop an identical generic summary form for every farm visit. Table 8.2 provides a framework to calculate the animal welfare status of each farm visited. It is based on calculating a single value for each of the five freedoms then developing an overall stock welfare index based on equal weightings of each of these five freedoms. This makes a value judgement that the five freedoms are of equal importance and so have equal impact on the cow's wellbeing. This assumption may require further discussion and feedback from some of the world's animal welfare experts. So Table 8.2 is a 'work in progress' but we believe it forms the basis of a relatively robust, yet quick, assessment of animal welfare on an individual small holder or large-scale farm.

Table 8.2. Calculation of an animal welfare index following a farm visit.

1. Freedom from hunger and thirst	
Total number of measures recorded (A); maximum of 7	
Sum of scores recorded (B)	
% score for Measure 1 (A/B x 100)	
2. Freedom from discomfort	
Total number of measures recorded (A); maximum of 8	
Sum of scores recorded (B)	
% score for Measure 2 (A/B x 100)	
3. Freedom from pain, injury and disease	
Total number of measures recorded (A); maximum, of 9	
Sum of scores recorded (B)	
% score for Measure 3 (A/B x 100)	
4. Freedom from fear and distress	
Total number of measures recorded (A); maximum of 5	
Sum of scores recorded (B)	
% score for Measure 4 (A/B x 100)	
5. Freedom to express normal behaviour	
Total number of measures recorded (A); maximum of 7	
Sum of scores recorded (B)	
% score for Measure 5 (A/B x 100)	
6. Farm animal welfare index	
Mean value of all five % above	

8.2 Case studies of dairy cow welfare

This section outlines two examples of how on-farm welfare has been measured using case studies. One example is in large European dairies, and the other in small African dairies. Both studies detail what recordings were taken and the conclusions made following the assessment of welfare. Together, they provide some examples of animal welfare issues likely to be found on Asian dairies and ways that they can be assessed.

8.2.1 Results from a UK study of dairy cow welfare indicators

Work by Whay *et al.* (2003) developed an on-farm scoring system for dairy cattle welfare. Measurements were chosen based on the 'five basic freedoms of animal welfare' and they collected data through both direct observations of animals and from farm records. A summary of the welfare measures used and the data collected is presented in Table 8.3. A total of 53 farms were studied and the results were divided into five bands, A to E, with the farms in the top 20% in band A and the worst scoring farms in band E. The allocation of a farm to a particular band was specific to each observation, and so each band would have contained different farms for each indicator.

There was a good association between levels of mastitis estimated by the producer and recorded incidences. This was not the case with lameness, however, with herd records for lameness being much lower than farmer perceptions, and farmer perceptions being much lower than levels of lameness scored in the on-farm assessment. (5.7 v 22.1%). These three sets of data have also been italicised in

Table 8.3. Results profile for welfare indicators on 53 dairy farms in United Kingdom. A, B, C, D and E refer to quintile bands of 20% of the farms.

	Unit	A	B	C	D	E
Production Annual milk yield	L/cow	8300–10 500	7789–8200	7118–7652	6500–7000	4275–6313
Nutrition						
Thin cows	%	0–6	6–11	13–21	22–31	33–62
Fat cows	%	0	0	0	1–6	5–28
Bloated rumen	%	0	3–6	7–17	18–24	25–47
Hollow rumen	%	0–6	7–14	14–21	21–31	32–82
Milk fever (Est) *	%/yr	0	0	0	1	1–31
Metabolic diseases (Est)	%/yr	0–3	3–4	5–7	7–9	10–19
Reproduction						
Conception to first service (Est)	%	68–80	60–66	56–59	49–55	28–48
Assisted calvings (Est)	%/yr	0	0	1	1–5	5–40
Disease						
Mastitis (Rec)	%/yr	0–9	11–21	21–34	41–46	47–120
Mastitis (Est)	%/yr	3–13	15–19	20–33	33–47	47–89
Lameness	%	0–14	14–18	20–23	24–30	31–50
Lameness (Rec)	%/yr	0	0	2–4	4–11	11–42
Lameness (Est)	%/yr	3–9	9–14	15–21	21–34	35–54
Claw overgrowth	%	0–12	12–25	27–34	35–46	46–76
Poor claw conformation	%	0	0	3–7	7–17	18–37
Dull/obviously sick	%	0	0	2–3	4–6	7–20
Sudden death/casualty (Est)	%/yr	0–1	1–2	2–3	3–4	4–16
External appearance						
Dirty hind limbs	%	65–85	90–96	97–100	100	100
Dirty udder	%	0–8	10–18	18–23	24–33	36–70
Dirty flanks	%	0	2–7	8–11	14–23	26–78
Hair loss	%	0	4–7	8–13	15–31	33–88
Environmental injury						
Hock hair loss	%	0–8	10–22	22–45	47–71	100
Swollen hock	%	0–11	11–28	29–36	37–68	70–97
Ulcerated hock	%	0	3–4	5–12	12–25	29–50
Non-hock injuries	%	6–43	46–59	59–66	67–79	80–100
Behaviour						
Average flight distance	m	0.6–1.1	1.2–1.5	1.5–1.7	1.7–1.9	2.1–3.4
Idle cows	%	0–3	3–4	5	6–8	8–25
Rising restrictions	%	0–10	12–20	30	33–40	50–78

*Est, estimated by the farmer; Rec, recorded by the farmer; all other data was observed by the research team during one visit.

Table 8.3. These results suggest that farmers are not detecting lameness, and this was highlighted as a major area where dairy cow welfare needed improving in the UK.

The research team also consulted experts to devise a threshold value, or a value at which experts believe action to address the issue should be taken. Whay *et al.* (2003) concluded that of the 53 farms, 32 needed to take action to reduce mastitis problems while 42 needed to actively reduce their feet and lameness problems. Furthermore, it was concluded that there were no consistently good or bad farms, rather that farms had different welfare strengths and weaknesses.

This experimental approach would have contributed to the formation of the protocols to measure welfare described above. This research could also be used as a blueprint to developing similar ways in small holder dairying to identify problem farms and second, to identify the farms with better stock welfare and herd performance.

8.2.2 Results from an African study highlighting poor cow welfare

Nguhiu-Mwangi *et al.* (2013) recently reported on a range of indicators of poor cow welfare on 112 SHD farms in Nairobi, Kenya. Like many Asian countries, the bulk (in this case 80%) of Kenya's domestic milk supplies originates from small holder farmers each with 2 to 20 zero-grazed milking cows. These small herds consist of mainly exotic European dairy breeds, making methods and results a useful point of comparison with Asian dairying systems.

The Kenyan study was directed towards two key aspects of welfare: first, the existence and degree of claw lesions, and second, body injuries, condition and body soiling. Both datasets were used to predict the welfare of zero-grazed dairy stock, accounting for different farm environments and management practices. While the study covered these aspects well, milk yields were not reported, and so an assessment of productivity was not performed.

A total of 300 cows, mainly Friesian crossbreds, on 32 farms were examined in the first study, following washing and trimming of their hind claws. For the second study, body condition, body soiling and signs of external body injuries were examined in additional 306 cows from 80 other farms. In both studies, herd sizes averaged 10, ranging from 5 to 20 milking cows, and a maximum of 5 cows per herd were examined.

In the first study, 88% of the 300 cows presented with claw lesions, of which 69% were subclinical and 31% were clinical through showing evidence of lameness. In the second study, 35% of the cows on 73% of the farms were clinically lame.

Superficial injuries to the neck were observed in cows on 65% of these farms. This was the result of poorly designed feeding areas, including low positioning of neck bars over the feed and excessive width of feed bunks. Other design issues with the feed bunk caused behavioural issues. Inadequate feeding space per animal often led to intensive competition and aggressive behaviour at feeding time. Very few of the feed bunks were concreted with many made of iron sheets and timber, and often with sharpened edges, which predisposed the cows to injuries in the mouth, head and neck areas.

Leg injuries, particularly of the front hocks (knees) were observed in 87% of the cows on 96% of the farms, while brisket injuries were observed in 44% of the cows on 64% of the farms. These were attributed to inadequate or no bedding in the stalls and the stalls simply being too small. Only 46% of the farms had any stall bedding, which varied from wheat straw, sawdust, wood shavings, plastic mats to bare wooden slats. In the remaining farms, cows either lay on dirt (53%) or concrete (47%). On 29% of the farms, the alleyways were not concreted, while in the concreted sheds, only 23% had good walking surfaces in which concrete was not too slippery or pitted with pot holes. Clearly hoof and leg health on many of these farms suffered due to the lack of soft, non-slip and washable floors with good drainage. In addition, the lack of comfortable bedding in the stalls discouraged the cows to lie down, this meant they had to endure long hours of standing in the alleyways.

Rib injuries were observed in 75% of the cows on 95% of the farms, as were hip injuries in 67% of the cows on 91% of the farms. Overstocking and poorly designed and maintained sheds were the major causes of these traumatic injuries. Teat, udder and thigh injuries were also prevalent, these being attributed to the roughness and bareness of the concrete floors and the stalls. The key predisposing factors to external body injuries clearly were the restrictiveness of housing types and the structures that affect cows' natural behaviour patterns. Even though the various injuries were the result of different risk factors, they were all due to the design, space and nature of the housing. With the key profit-driven objective of producing more milk, many of these farmers increased the size of their existing sheds or simply housed more cows. In both cases, without better strategic planning, cow welfare clearly suffered.

Low neck bars and high bunks in the feeding area increased the number of neck and brisket injuries, narrow alleyways increased hock injuries and poor quality, rough and pot-holed concrete floors increased the hip injuries. Teat, udder and thigh injuries all increased on farms where no bedding was provided. Lameness was closely associated with the quality of effluent management, such as the amount of slurry on alleyways. Small cubicles and overstocked sheds restricted movements and the expression of normal behaviour.

Cow body condition indicated moderate quality feeding management with very few cows being either too fat or too thin. Increasing the frequency and amount of concentrate feeding, mineral and protein supplements led to improved body condition scores. Surprisingly, 15% of the farmers did not feed concentrates at all, depending entirely on harvested forage to supply the nutrient requirements of their milking cows. The forages ranged from Napier (*Pennisetum purpureum*), Kikuyu (*Pennisetum clandestinum*) and Rhodes grasses (*Chloris gayana*) and maize stover and occasionally banana plant stems. Concentrates were mainly commercially formulated (99%), fed mainly to the milking cows only (on 84% of the farms) with farmers feeding an enormous range in daily amounts; 32% fed from 2 to 4 kg, 29% fed from 5 to 7 kg, 24% fed from 8 to 10 kg while 14% more than 10 kg/cow/day. Mineral supplements were commonly fed (on 89% of the farms) whereas protein supplements were only fed on 36% of the farms.

Cow cleanliness was not good in that 97% of the cows had flank soiling and 90% had soiled udders. Only 55% of the farms removed slurry and cleaned and hosed down concrete floors each day. Cow cleanliness was closely associated with shed hygiene. Only 76% of the cows were milked outside their resting area, often in unsuitable improvised stalls. Only 12% of the farms had specific maternity stalls.

One of the more disappointing findings in this study was that farmers had very poor perceptions of cow welfare. Although across the two studies 99% and 89% of them agreed that milking cows should have ready access to feed and water, respectively, this was not always provided. Only 47% agreed on the need to alleviate unnecessary pain with prompt medical attention while just 25% shared the opinion that animals suffer when mistreated and they should be protected from conditions exposing them to distress. Only 29% considered that there was a need for good shelter and housing systems to avoid discomfort and physical stress while just 5% agreed to the need to provide sufficient housing space with adequate facilities to allow expression of normal behaviour patterns. The farmers and stockpeople also had poor human–animal interactions with shouting and whipping of cows commonly recorded.

In conclusion, substandard housing design, poor husbandry practices and farmer ignorance were the key factors leading to the poor cow welfare on these farms. Being aware of these issues is the first step to improving welfare.

9

Stock management on Asian small holder dairy farms

This chapter discusses the management of South East Asian small holder dairy (SHD) farms highlighting the key constraints to cow performance and how these impact on cow welfare.

The main points of this chapter

- In far too many cases, SHD farmers develop their production systems based on the 'traditional way of doing things'. Such farm management decisions and practices are based on how their father, friends or neighbour does things, together with their own trial and error experiences and some advice from service providers.
- Grazed forages provide only a negligible proportion of the stockfeed on SHD farms in the tropics. Some of the reasons for this are listed in this chapter.
- The short answer to the question of why cows are zero grazed in the tropics is the combination of high land costs and cheap labour.
- In many tropical Asian countries, considerable attention has been given to cow colonies, which consist of large dairy sheds, holding 50 or more cows that are owned by a number of SHD farmers. The perceived benefits of cow colonies lie in the economies of scale the farmers are hoping from the total herd management. Such an approach can overcome many constraints to production but may introduce others.

- On any dairy farm, no matter its size or location, the dairy production technology can be broken down into nine key activities, which can be considered as steps in the supply chain of profitable dairy farming. Just as any chain is only as strong as its weakest link, each step in this supply chain must be properly managed.
- Within a list of 34 key on-farm constraints to milk production technology on tropical SHD farms, the majority (26 of them) have implications for animal welfare. There is a close association between profitable farming and good animal welfare. This highlights the importance of understanding the necessity of, and practising, good animal welfare to improve farm performance, profitability and sustainability.
- The average milk production of all lactating cows in the herd can provide a useful guide as to the adequacy of the current dairy farm management practices. On tropical SHD farms, this can vary from less than 5 to more than 20 kg/cow/d due to genetics, feeding management and other farm factors.
- An assessment was made of the comparative performance of 15 SHD farms in the humid tropics, half in the lowlands and the rest in the highlands of the same dairy region in SE Asia. The striking difference was their average daily milk production, 8.3 (lowlands) v 13.5 (highlands) kg/cow/day. This could be attributed to climatic stress, herd and feeding management which impinged on their animal welfare.
- A study of 30 dairy farms in Peninsula Malaysia provided many valuable insights into why some farms are productive and profitable and why others are not. In essence, higher per cow milk yields and farm profitabilities were recorded on farms that were better equipped and better managed.
- This chapter contains a checklist of current farm management and stock welfare observations to assess the performance and likely profitability of the farm.

9.1 Dairy farming in the developing tropics

Globally, agriculture provides a livelihood for more people than any other industry (primary or secondary) while dairy farming is one of these major agricultural activities. In fact, Hemme and Otto (2010) estimated that 12 to 14% of the world's population (or 750 to 900 million people) live on dairy farms or within dairy farming households. Livestock provide over half the value of global agricultural output and one-third of this is in developing countries. Growth in agricultural production and productivity is then needed to raise rural incomes and to meet the food and raw material needs of the faster-growing urban populations. Because livestock products are more costly than other staple foods, their consumption levels are still low in these countries, although they are increasing as incomes rise. Milk is nature's most complete food and dairy farming represents one of the fastest returns for livestock keepers in the developing world. Furthermore, increased dairy production and greater self-sufficiency save on foreign exchange.

Milk is a cash crop for small holders, converting low value forages and crop residues, and using family labour, into a valued market commodity. The dairy industry occupies a unique position among other sectors of agriculture as it gives a regular income to farmers due to milk being produced every day. Furthermore, milk production is highly labour intensive, providing a lot of employment. Accordingly, SHD farming was established as part of social welfare and rural development schemes throughout the developing tropics to supply a regular cash flow for poorly resourced and often-landless farmers. It now provides regular income to farmers, especially to women, enhances household nutrition and food security and creates off-farm employment. As many as one job is created for each 20 kg milk processed and marketed (Hooten 2008). The development of SHD also addresses the opportunities to overcome the persistent problem of rural poverty. This is by transferring income from affluent urban households to their poorer rural counterparts as well as improving the food and nutritional security for poor rural and urban households.

In many developing countries, the availability of meat and milk improves the level of human nutrition. These sectors are largely produced from land that is unsuitable for cropping, and utilises agro-industrial by-products that would otherwise be expensive to dispose of – such as straw. In addition, cattle farming provides draught power, meaningful employment for some of the poorest members of the community and also can provide them with dung, a useful source of fuel to reduce reliance on wood and fossil fuels.

The advantages of integrating dairy production in crop systems offer great potential. This is because, compared to pastoralists and agro-pastoralists, these farmers have more control over feed inputs and are able to capture complementarities in feed resource use and nutrient recycling, which increase overall farm efficiency and reduce vulnerability to market shifts. These crop–livestock systems generally support higher rural population densities than other solely livestock systems.

Unlike other tropical regions, milk from cattle, buffaloes and goats is not a traditional component of diets in South-East (SE) Asia. Rather, the milk they consumed came from coconuts, not livestock. Only over the last few decades has there has been increasing interest in dairying throughout this region. Higher population pressures and changes in eating habits have increased the demand for dairy products. Many countries now have school milk programs to encourage young children to drink more milk and hence improve their health through increased consumption of energy, protein and minerals (particularly calcium and phosphorus). In future years, as these children grow and have families, milk consumption will increase at a faster rate. Consequently, many SE Asian countries are striving towards self-sufficiency in dairy products, at least in drinking milk.

The demand for milk in SE Asia is expected to continue increasing well into the future, driven by population growth and affluence. Per capita consumption is rising fastest in regions where rapid income growth and urbanisation result in people adding variety to their diets. Because of the relatively high cost of handling perishable final products and taste factors, most of this milk will be produced where it is consumed, aided by increasing imports of feed grains.

Now SHD is an accepted rural industry in virtually every tropical country in the world. The climatic, soil and socio economic environments of the tropics have created a very different type of industry to that found in the temperate developed countries and this is the subject of this chapter. It discusses the current systems of managing SHD farms in tropical Asia and their implications with stock behaviour and welfare.

Table 1.1 in Chapter 1 lists the Asian countries with low self-sufficiencies of, hence large imports of, milk and dairy products. These countries all have active programs to import dairy heifers to increase their national dairy herd populations. It is apparent that many of these countries do not have the same knowledge of how to manage high producing dairy cows as exporting countries, and so this leads to significant welfare concerns.

This chapter essentially discusses the limitations of traditional management and how, in too many cases, SHD farmers are developing their production systems based on the 'traditional way of doing things'. Tradition is a generic word used in this case to mean basing farm management decisions and practices on how their father, or friends or even nextdoor neighbour does things. This is complementary with their own trial and error experiences and maybe some advice from service providers, such as dairy cooperative or government advisers. Rarely do SHD farmers take full advantage of all the information sources available to them, with many of them available for free. As reported in the African small holder farmer case study in Chapter 8.2.2, farmer ignorance is a common cause of cow welfare problems in the developing tropics.

9.2 Shedding dairy stock in tropical Asia

9.2.1 Why are dairy stock generally housed in tropical Asia?

Grazed forages provide only a negligible (often zero) proportion of the stockfeed on SHD farms in the tropics for a wide variety of reasons, as listed below. However, the short answer to the question of why cows are zero grazed in the tropics is due to the combination of high land costs and cheap labour.

- High population pressures provide considerable competition for land, hence it is expensive to purchase or rent.

- Labour costs are low, therefore the use of machinery to harvest forages is minimal and forages are commonly harvested by hand on most SHD farms.
- Maintaining forage quality through grazing management is more difficult with tropical forages, compared to slower growing temperate forage species, so its regular harvesting and fertilising are best undertaken by humans at predetermined intervals rather than by livestock.
- Forage can be more easily hand harvested from erect, rather than prostrate, forage species that are fast growing and so more productive in the hot and humid climates of the tropics.
- The efficiency of removing all the forage from the pasture is invariably greater using a hand-held machete (or sickle) or a mechanical brush cutter than could possibly be achieved by a grazing animal that selectively chooses the most palatable parts of the forage and frequently defecates and urinates on other parts of the sward.
- The high temperatures and humidities encountered in the tropics necessitate the provision of shade, controlled ventilation (through shed designs and occasional fans) and water cooling (using hoses or sprinkler systems) which is best provided in sheds, preferably with open sides.
- Shedding provides weather proofing against climatic extremes, such as monsoonal rains which upset stock and SHD management routines such as herding grazing stock twice daily for milking.
- Security, particularly biosecurity, can be a major concern, both from people who can steal stock from open pastures and from other livestock that can spread contagious diseases.
- It makes tick and other parasite control easier.

These benefits of 100% shedding of stock are offset by the extra labour required to harvest the forages and to clean and maintain the shed facilities. The other problem is that shedding removes the opportunity for the cows' to graze and so express the associated normal behaviour arising from the freedom to move around and socialise in relatively large areas. Welfare issues are more likely to arise in the confinements of a shed than out at pasture. Animal health issues would be less prevalent at pasture with its healthier environment (hence lower exposure to pathogens) and greater opportunity for stock to move around, interact with each other and relax in the open air. The only extra precaution needed would be to more closely monitor and control parasites (external and internal) to prevent them rapidly infesting the stock once housed. Intakes of forage by grazing stock are also harder to monitor than if they were in the shed, making ration formulation more difficult.

If the opportunity arises, weaned heifers or non-lactating cows would be the easiest to put out to graze as they do not require the closer daily attention of milk-fed calves and milking cows.

9.2.2 Problems of confinement

Dairy stock imported from Western countries have almost invariably been reared under grazing conditions, and therefore have never been exposed to a continual shed environment, as is common on most tropical SHD farms. Compared to grazing, confinement creates specific problems such as:

- Restricting opportunity to seek comfort, for example, if they are only provided with cement floors.
- Physical problems related to continuously lying on cement, such as bed sores and ulcers, inflamed and infected joints (arthritis) and muscle damage causing pain.
- Creating problems of high humidity in poorly ventilated sheds, that can be just as detrimental as high temperatures.
- Limiting opportunity for exercise, hence the need for routine hoof trimming.
- Increasing exposure to infectious diseases.
- Other health issues, such as mastitis and uterine infections when hygiene is poor during milking and calving.
- Creating problems of heat detection for artificial insemination in the confinements of a shed.
- Requiring greater efforts to ensure good sanitation.
- Magnifying problems of social dominance in the herd.
- Often upsetting natural behaviour patterns.
- Increasing capital investment.

9.2.3 Potential role for cow colonies

In many tropical Asian countries, considerable attention has been given to large-scale investments in 'cow colonies'. These consist of large dairy sheds, holding 50 or more cows that are owned by several SHD farmers. These are generally located in close proximity to areas of forage production. Although small holders still own and manage their own herds in these large sheds, the perceived benefits of cow colonies lie in the larger size of the total herd and shared management costs. Such an approach can overcome many constraints to production, but may introduce others as listed below:

Potential benefits of cow colonies

- Greater investment potential since cooperatives have more borrowing power than individual farmers
- Use of mechanical forage choppers and milking machines
- Can employ contract labour to rear young stock
- Can grow large areas for forages, such as maize, for livestock feeding
- Less wastage in recycling manure to forage production area, through building effluent ponds to minimise volatilisation of nitrogen from urine

- Bulk handling of conserved forages using large-scale silage ensiling and storage systems
- Easier communication between advisers and farmers and between farmers themselves
- Easier to implement training programs involving practical skills as well as technical theory
- Easier to monitor post-training the application of new skills
- Better motivation of farmers to improve management practices as they can more easily observe such benefits
- Easier monitoring of individual farmer's milking hygiene practices and hence individual remuneration for better quality milk
- Concentrating farmers in the one place provides an ideal opportunity to introduce other motivation techniques such as regular awards for best management practices
- Better coordination of forage production, cow feeding, insemination, animal health, milk handling etc.
- Upskilling of farmers in specialist skills such as machine milking or calf rearing so they can take over much of these responsibilities in cow colonies
- Installation of milk cooling units on site
- More rapid cooling of milk and greater availability of hot water for more effective cleaning and sanitising equipment
- Increased likelihood of sufficient milk production to justify small value-adding operations to benefit small dairy cooperatives
- Greater potential returns to the local dairy cooperative, and so to the farmers themselves.

Unfortunately, such impressive facilities go hand in hand with high profile projects such as stocking them with imported pregnant Friesian heifers. The high mortality rates all too often experienced in these tropical countries suggest that the current colony feeding and herd management has yet to be improved to an appropriate level to achieve many of the production benefits from these high genetic merit animals. Also, animals with genetics more suitable to the conditions should be utilised, with the long-term higher productivity gains being weighed up against short-term production reduction. This would also result in more desirable welfare, and farmer satisfaction outcomes.

Potential problems with cow colonies
- Sheds are constructed and filled with cows before the forage production area has been developed, leading to many poorly fed cows.
- Insufficient attention is given to growing out non-revenue generating, young stock.

- Poorly planned forage production areas, e.g. with minimal water for irrigation during the dry season.
- Insufficient land allocated to forage production, partly because of provision of insufficient daily forage allocations to achieve more realistic target milk yields.
- Incorrect perception that rice straw, sugarcane tops and over mature maize stover are suitable forage sources for milking cows, particularly when target milk yields are 15 L/cow/day or more (Moran 2014).
- Lack of understanding of the potential of quality forages and tree legumes as important roughage sources for high yielding cows.
- Potential spread of disease because of variable management between individual farmers, e.g. during calf rearing, mastitis – if using milking machines.
- Poor concept of the need for more sophisticated milking hygiene when using milking machines, e.g. regular replacing of milk liners and testing of machine performance.
- Continual breakdown of machinery, choppers and milking machines.
- Need for highly trained and well-skilled labour for year round supply of quality forages.
- Need for senior managers to develop both short-term and long-term views on development program.
- Difficulties of regularly sourcing finances for completion of these large-scale capital development projects, such as provision of milking equipment, durable forage choppers.
- Inherent problems of passing over responsibility to individuals within small management teams. The larger the operation the more essential it is that skilled individuals be given more responsibility in specialist areas, such as forage production, animal health, milk quality.
- Management teams for large-scale cow colonies should not be expected to oversee those of any nearby small holder farms.
- Need for senior managers to find and keep quality staff with capabilities of solving both day-to-day small management problems as well as contribute to large-scale development. This problem could be addressed by employing bright, practically minded young animal science graduates who would be prepared to live as well as work in villages near cow colonies.
- With the penalties imposed by milk processors, returns on these large capital investments are markedly reduced because of the low unit milk returns through poor quality milk. Small investments, such as steam cleaners, small hot water units become even more effective in light of the large capital costs of sheds, silage bunkers etc.
- As with all small holder ventures, it is more profitable to 'feed fewer cows better'.

Poorly resourced SHD farmers, whose businesses are often in 'survival mode', can become very individualistic and take time to develop the cooperative, sharing nature required for successful cow colonies. This has been given as a common reason for their poor success rate in countries with relatively new SHD industries such as Indonesia. However, small holders in countries like China, which have more of a history of collective farming, utilise these benefits of magnitude of scale, particularly with some of their specific farm operations such as preserving and storing large amounts of silage and sharing a milking parlour so it can operate more efficiently for many hours of each day and night.

9.3 Constraints to farm performance and profitability

9.3.1 Supply chain for profitable dairy farming

On any dairy farm, no matter its size or location, the dairy production technology can be broken down into nine key on-farm activities, that can be considered as steps in the supply chain of profitable dairy farming (Moran 2009a). Just as any chain is only as strong as its weakest link, each step in this supply chain must be properly managed. Weakening any one link through poor decision-making and farming practices can have severe ramifications on overall farm performance and hence profits. In chronological order of their role in ensuring a profitable dairy enterprise, the 'links' are presented in Figure 9.1. Of these 9 steps, numbers 2, 3, 4, 5, 6 and 7 would all have implications for animal welfare.

9.3.2 Identifying the key constraints to animal welfare within the supply chain

The dairy industries of tropical Asia have failed to keep pace with the speed of dairy development in Western countries over recent decades. Granted, the tropical environment is not ideal for dairy cows as high temperatures and humidities and seasonal rainfall reduce both the nutritive value of available forages and the level of cow comfort, that is the production potential and welfare of the stock. In addition, many of the farmers, usually small holders with less than 10 milking cows, have not been able to develop the skills of efficient milk production. This has primarily been due to poor extension services more so than lack of technical knowledge on tropical dairy farming. Constraints to profitable dairy farming in tropical Asia are many and varied and can be categorised into institutional, government, socio-economic, technical and post-farm gate.

Within the technical constraints, Moran (2013) identified 34 key on-farm constraints to milk production technology, based on their position in the supply chain. An extra category 'Other on-farm constraints' is included in the following tables to take into account those skills covering farm business management. The ones with direct implications for animal welfare are presented in Table 9.1 while

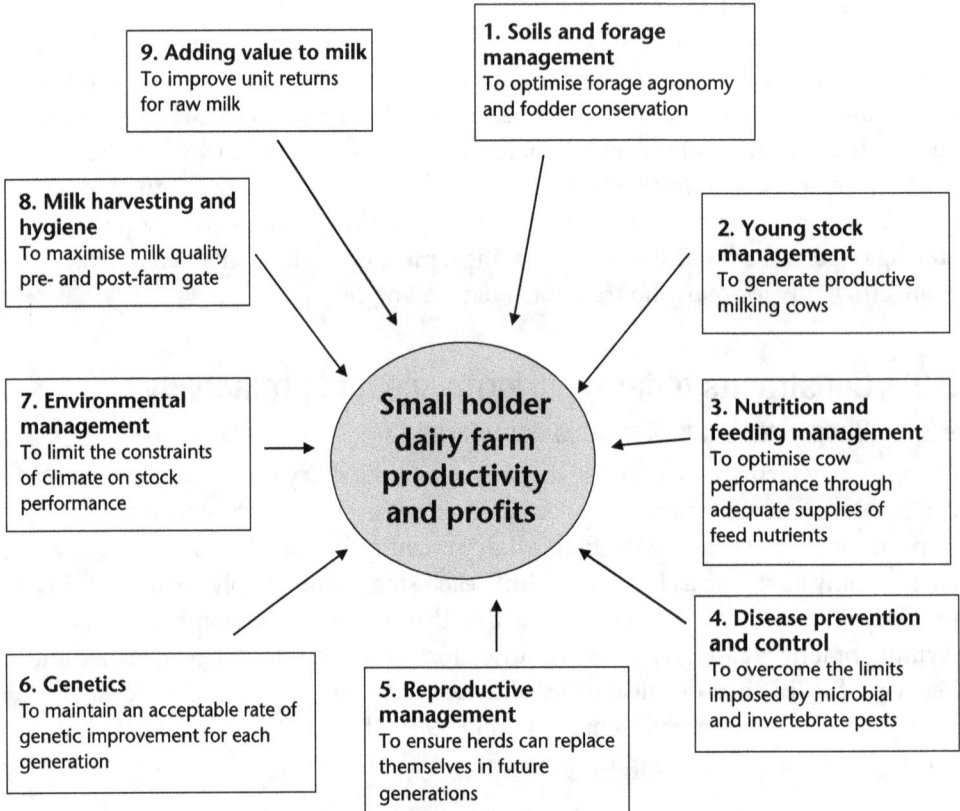

Figure 9.1: The nine steps in the on-farm supply chain of profitable dairy farming.

those with little or no direct implications for animal welfare are presented in Table 9.2.

From Table 9.1, 26 of the 34 constraints have implications for animal welfare, while the remaining constraints (listed in Table 9.2) could be considered to have little or no direct implications. The only ones without implications for animal welfare were those related to milk quality and unit returns, increasing the proportion of heifer calves in the herd, collecting robust herd performance data and improving farmer–management dairy co-op relationships. In other words, the majority of farm management decisions and practices would impinge on animal welfare issues. This highlights the significance of understanding the importance of, and practising, good animal welfare to improve farm performance, profitability and sustainability. We would expect that in any region of tropical Asia, or in fact in any dairying region around the world, there would be a close correlation between profitable and sustainable farms and good animal welfare practices. In other words, not only is sound animal welfare essential from the cows' contented

Table 9.1. On-farm constraints to milk production technology (from Moran 2013) with direct implications for animal welfare.

Key activity	Key constraints with implications for animal welfare
1. Soils and forage management	Shortage of dry season forages
2. Young stock management	High calf mortality Poor post weaning growth rates High wastage rates (from birth to conceiving in 2nd lactation)
3. Nutrition and feeding management	Low quality of by-products and formulated concentrates Poor performance of cows during early lactation (poor peak and daily milk yields, delayed cycling) Cows (particularly high genetic merit cows) do not cycle for many weeks after calving Seasonality of milk production Little profits in milking cows
4. Disease prevention and management	Problems with lameness Problems with mastitis High calf and heifer morbidity and mortality General animal health problems
5. Reproductive management	High age at first calving Low 100 day in calf rate (pregnant within 100 days from calving) or high 200 not in calf rate (not pregnant within 200 days of calving) High number of services per conception Low % mature cows are milking
6. Genetics	Poor milking cow quality Most suitable genotype for the system
7. Environmental management	High incidence of heat stress during the 24 h period High incidence of animal health problems due to poor shed hygiene
8. Milk harvesting management	Poor milk composition (fat and protein contents)
9. Value adding milk	–
10. Other on farm constraints	Poor profitability of dairy farming Low capital resources for investing in farm infrastructure Poor dairy farming skills Underdeveloped entrepreneurial skills in dairy farmers

existence and hence the farmers' ethical viewpoint, it is also an essential ingredient of the farmers' smorgasbord to ensure a long-term and profitable future.

9.3.3 Farm Key Performance Indicators and animal welfare

Moran (2009b) developed a range of Key Performance Indicators (KPI) to help farmers diagnose the strengths and weaknesses in their dairy enterprise. Table 9.3 presents 10 questions that should be asked on any farm, big or small. The full paper presents the relevant values for each question. The first six, being feed related, have few implications for animal welfare, apart from the need to ensure the stock have sufficient forage supplies to ensure normal rumen function and that their appetites

Table 9.2. On farm constraints to milk production technology (from Moran 2013) with little or no direct implications for animal welfare.

Key activity	Key constraints with little or no implications for animal welfare
1. Soils and forage management	Low yields of forage Poor forage quality
2. Young stock management	–
3. Nutrition and feeding management	–
4. Disease prevention and management	–
5. Reproductive management	Increasing the proportion of heifer calves
6. Genetics	Difficulty of collecting robust data from genetic improvement programs
7. Environmental management	Reduced forage quality due to high temperatures and rainfall
8. Milk harvesting management	Poor milk quality (bacterial contamination)
9. Value adding milk	Poor milk unit returns
10. Other on-farm constraints	Poor farmer–management dairy co-op relationships

Table 9.3. Ten KPIs of small holder dairy farm performance.

Measure	Questions to ask
Feeding management	
1. Stocking capacity	Is the farm carrying too many cattle for the available forage supplies?
2. On farm forage production	How much of the farm's annual forage requirements must be purchased?
3. Forage quality	Is the forage being harvested or purchased at its optimal quality for milking cows?
4. Concentrate feeding program	What is the quality of the concentrates being fed and how much is allocated per milking cow?
5. Total feed costs	Are the forages and concentrates costing too much per unit of feed energy or protein?
6. Milk income less feed costs	How does this compare with those of other farmers with good feeding management?
Herd management	
7. Percentage productive cows	What is the percentage of adult cows actually milking? What is the proportion of milking cows in the entire dairy herd, expressed as a percentage?
8. Pattern of milk production	What is the peak milk yield of the herd and what is its lactation persistency (rate of decline from peak milk yield)?
9. Reproductive performance	How many days after calving do cows cycle? What is the submission rate and the conception rate to first insemination?
10. Heifer management	What are the pre-weaning calf mortality and the wastage rate of heifers from birth to second lactation? What is their age and live weight at first calving?

are not adversely affected by poor cow comfort. However, the remaining four are all directly affected by poor animal welfare practices.

One of the major problems on tropical small holder farms is the high calf mortality and the very high ages at first calving of replacement heifers. Pre-weaning calf mortality rates of 15 to 25% would be typical on many tropical dairy farms (Moran 2011) and can be as high as 50%; this contrasts to the 3 to 5% mortality rates on farms in temperate developed countries. Ages at first calving vary from 30 to 36 months on most tropical SHD farms, compared the 24 to 30 month targets. These clearly indicate poor calf and heifer rearing practices. Many of these are due to poor stock welfare, such as inadequate housing and hygiene, which exaggerate the other shortfalls in feeding and disease management. This again highlights one of the main themes of this book that improving welfare will lead to production and productivity improvements.

9.3.4 Assessing adequacy of the current herd management using cow milk yields

All the above KPIs can be quantified to provide guidelines as to which ones require priority in any dairy farm improvement program. Although some are relatively easy to quantify, others are quite difficult. Probably the most simple, and most used, single measure of SHD farm performance is the average milk yield of the milking cows. The correct term for this figure is 'rolling herd average' as it is the average milk yield of all the lactating cows, which will be at various stages in their lactation cycle.

This single value provides a summation of all the important aspects of SHD farm management, so any interpretation must take into account a diversity of feeding, herd and farm factors. Accordingly, many dairy specialists may query its usefulness as a single measure of dairy farm performance. However, it is routinely used by farmers to describe their farm's performance in relation to their neighbour's farm and also in relation to production targets provided by many government advisers. In addition, it is often quoted by government officials when summarising the stage of development of their national dairy industries. Table 9.4 describes the adequacy of the farm's dairy farm management practices using the rolling herd average; other factors to consider are listed below the table (see also Figures 9.2 and 9.3).

Other factors to consider

- It is important to differentiate between rolling herd averages and peak milk yields
- Milk composition is also a good indicator of feeding management
- Excessive body condition is indicative of nutrient status

Table 9.4. Interpreting the adequacy of dairy farm management from cow milk yields.

Range in average herd milk yields on tropical South-East Asian dairy farms

Herd milk yield (kg/cow/day)	Adequacy of dairy farm management practices
5 7	Very poor feeding and herd management and low genetic merit cows (or milking buffalo)
9	Typical of many SE Asian small holder farms, even with high grade Friesians
11 13 15 17 19	Gradual response with grade and crossbred Friesian cows to improved feeding, herd, young stock and shed management. *Milk yields of 15 kg/day are considered acceptable by many government dairy advisers.*
20	Potential level in **lowland humid tropics** following improved management of body condition throughout lactation
25	High genetic merit cows in **tropical highlands** or **lowland dry tropics** with good farm management
30	Typical peak milk yields in herds with 25 kg/cow/day rolling herd averages
35	Unrealistic in SE Asia except where all major constraints to milk production have been overcome

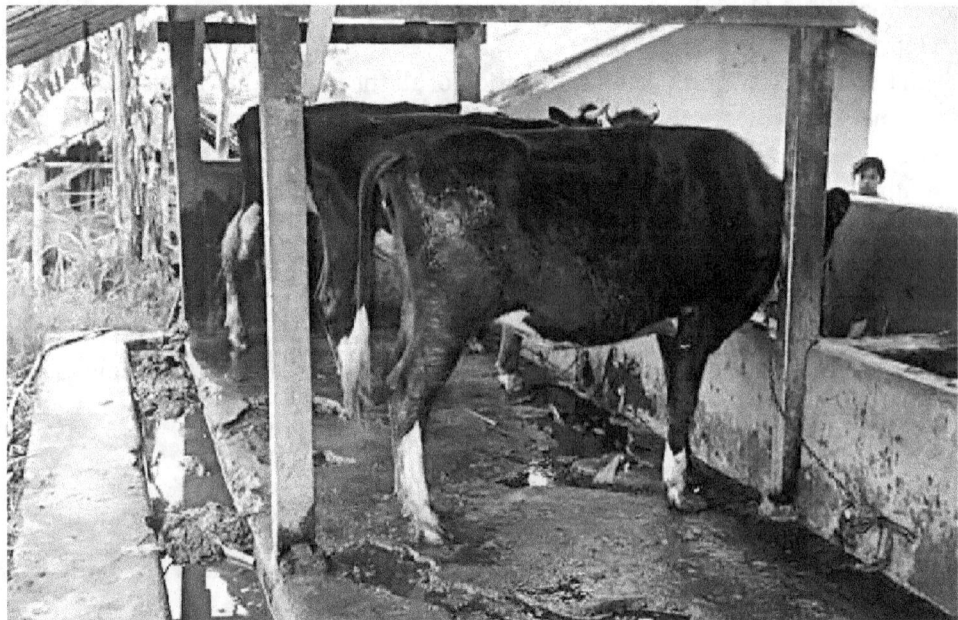

Figure 9.2: Typical housing system for tropical small holder dairy farmers; tie stall and concrete floor with very poor floor hygiene.

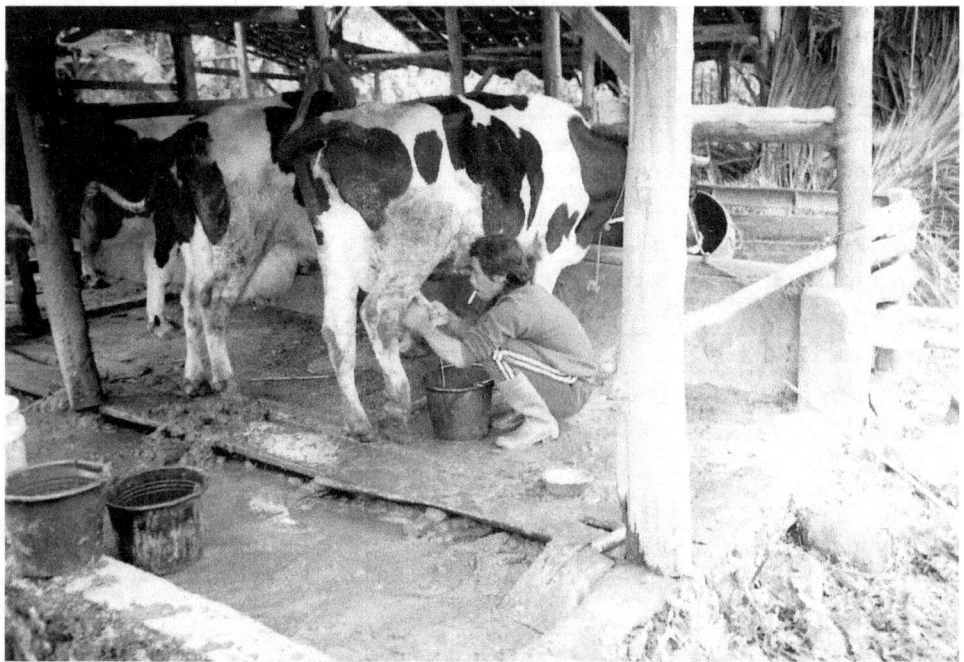

Figure 9.3: Permanently tethering milking cows that are maintained in very unhygienic conditions like this, could not be expected to produce much quality milk.

- Herd dynamics (number of dry cows and percentage of lactating adult cows in the herd) can also indicate adequacy of herd management.

9.3.5 Case study of small holder dairy farming in Indonesia

The adequacy of dairy farm management was assessed on a brief visit to a dairy farming region in the humid tropics of Indonesia during March 2013 where many SHD farms were located, some in the lowlands (at sea level) and others in the highlands (up to 1000 m above sea level). The milking cows were all crossbred Friesian and were tethered all day. The forage was essentially Napier grass (*Pennisetum purpureum*) or native grass sourced from the roadside or paddy fields while the concentrates were formulated commercially and supplemented with by-products from soy and cassava processing. The only drinking water offered to the cows was in the slurry mixed with the concentrates. There was no evidence of fans or water used to cool the cows on any of the farms. The temperature and humidity were recorded inside each cowshed and farmers were asked about their feeding management and cow milk yields. Local dairy advisers provided more information about the background of the farmers. The data and subjective assessments collected from these visits are presented in Table 9.5.

Table 9.5. Comparative performance of 8 lowland and 7 highland SHD farms in Indonesia.

	Lowland	Highland
Temperature in shed (°C)	31–33	26–30
Temperature Humidity Index in shed*	81–85	74–79
Milking cows per farm (range and av)	7–35, 16	1–7, 3
Range in farm milk yield (kg/cow/d)	6–11	8–16
Average farm milk yield (kg/cow/d)	**8.3**	**13.5**
Range in farm peak milk yield (kg/cow/d)	10–14	16–25
Forage sources	Roadside	Production areas/roadside
Forage quality	Poor to average	Average to good
Sheds	Densely populated, low roofs	Less densely populated, higher roofs
Drinking water	Slurry	Slurry
Natural ventilation	Poor	Better
Rubber mats	Very few	More
Shed hygiene	Not good	Better
Farmers	Conservative	More progressive
Cow body condition	Not good	Better
Stock welfare	Not good	Better

*Temperature Humidity Index, the higher the more heat stress, 78–89 is severe stress.

The lowland farms suffered from more severe heat stress and the cows were more poorly fed and managed than those on the highland farms. The sheds there provided better housing conditions and natural ventilation and there were more rubber mats per cow in the highland farms while the level of cow hygiene and the body condition of the cows was also better. The striking difference between the two areas was the higher daily average milk yield, 8.3 compared with 13.5 kg/cow/d for the lowland and highland farms respectively.

Clearly the difference in level of climatic stress and the herd, feeding management and welfare accounted for 5.2 kg/cow/d difference in the milk yields of farms in the two regions. The smaller size of highland herds would also have contributed to their better level of management and stock welfare.

9.3.6 Case study of small holder dairy farming in Malaysia

Farm production and business performance data were collected from 30 dairy farms in Peninsula Malaysia during September 2012 by Moran and Brouwer (2013). Observations of the stock, cowshed, farm facilities and forage production area were made to assess current farm practices and the general state of the stock and the supporting dairy infrastructure. Farmers were interviewed about key aspects of their farm management, the costs of farm inputs and their herd performance to develop a series of Key Performance Indicators. The business focus covered specific aspects of milk returns and feeding management to calculate total feed costs, feed efficiencies and feeding profits. Gross farm profits were calculated, including and excluding imputed labour costs. The farms were split into three groups to assess the impacts of farm management on cow milk yields. The key data findings are summarised in Table 9.6.

Herds with higher average milk yields contained a greater proportion of adult cows and replacement heifers. The milking cows had higher feed intakes and higher ration quality while the cows had higher feed efficiencies in that they converted more of their feed into saleable milk. Even though the farmers spent more money on feeding their milking cows better, these more productive herds yielded greater feeding profits from milk sales and they had lower costs of unit milk production. As these cows increased their milk production, the efficiency with which these farmers utilised their farm assets (both gross assets and assets that they actually owned) also increased.

The survey provided many valuable insights into why some farms are productive and profitable and why others are not. In essence, higher per cow milk yields and farm profitabilities were recorded on farms that were better equipped

Table 9.6. The impact of herd average daily milk yield on farm performance and business data of 30 farms in Peninsular Malaysia. The farms are grouped into either A, B or C (10 farms per group) based on increasing per cow milk yields.

Farm data	A	B	C	Sig
Herd average daily milk yield (kg/cow/d)	7.5	9.7	12.4	*
Size of milking herd (cows)	22	48	27	
% milking cows in adult herd	49	53	61	
% replacement heifers	47	73	80	*
Dry matter intake (kg/cow/d)	10.8	12.4	14.6	*
Ration metabolisable energy content (MJ//kg DM)	8.1	8.5	9.0	*
Ration crude protein content (%)	11.6	12.1	12.3	
Feed conversion efficiency (kg DM/kg milk)	0.70	0.82	0.87	*
Total feed costs for milkers (RM/cow/d)	7.44	8.75	11.41	*
Total feed costs as % milk income	78	76	49	*
Milk income less feed costs for entire herd (RM/kg milk)	0.53	0.57	1.24	*
Gross farm profit (RM/kg milk)	−2.01	−0.75	−0.05	*
Cost of production (RM/kg milk)	4.77	3.53	2.82	*
Feed costs (% total farm costs)	38	40	43	
Return on assets (%)	−0.6	−0.4	0.1	*
Return on equity (%)	−0.9	−0.5	0.1	*

* Significant difference between herds; RM, Malaysian ringgits.

and better managed resulting in better welfare. The more productive and profitable farmers had more reliable electricity and water supplies, provided specific calving down areas, did not graze their milking cows and did not suckle their calves on milkers. In addition, they used artificial insemination rather than natural mating, used calf milk replacer as part of their milk rearing program, routinely used dry cow therapy as part of the mastitis control program, kept farm records and had fewer problems with mastitis, lameness and young stock rearing. More of the cows on the most profitable farms had high peak milk yields and fewer had short lactations. Although these farmers invested more in feeding for their milking cows, the resultant greater feed conversion efficiencies on these farms and resultant better animal welfare yielded higher feeding profits and higher returns on total farm assets and equities.

Cowshed designs were generally poor in that roofs were low, shed hygiene had much that could be improved and fans and cooling sprinkler systems were virtually non-existent on any of the 30 farms. In addition, many of the farms suffered from a lack of productive cows in their herds. Future herd management must concentrate on improving reproductive performance and, in some instances, reducing young stock mortality as well as improving the nutritional status and therefore performance of the milking herd. Of the 30 farms surveyed, only eight had positive gross farm profits, although this increased to 18 farms if farmers excluded their family labour from the costs of milk production.

9.4 Checklist to assess current farm management and herd welfare

A series of observations can easily be made when visiting any dairy farm to assess the management and welfare of the stock and the performance and likely profitability of the farm. Answers to a series of questions could also be sought to help understand the current farm management. The following checklist has also been presented as Appendix 2.

Shed and facilities
- Roof height and natural ventilation
- Temperature and humidity inside shed
- Shed floor and cow lying area (cement, mats)
- Mats, enough for all cows, thin v thick
- Other forms of bedding material
- Stalls; tie stalls v free stalls v open lot
- General stocking density and space for cows to rest
- Adequacy and cleanliness of pens for young stock (heifers, milk-fed calves)
- Area for outside resting at night

- Adequacy and cleanliness of feed troughs and water containers
- Access to clean drinking water, not only as slurry feeding
- Source and adequacy of water for drinking and cleaning
- If sufficient cows, use of mechanical forage chopper
- Room for feed processing and preparation
- Adequacy and hygiene of milking area, including teat dipping and access to hot water
- If machine milking, state of rubber linings
- Cleanliness of milking buckets and milk cans
- General hygiene and condition of cow teats and coats
- Adequacy of effluent disposal and storage system
- Adequacy of office and farm staff area

Stock
- General condition (thin v good v fat)
- Obvious health issues, such as lameness
- Freedom from obvious injuries
- Is mastitis an issue? If so, what are the management procedures?
- Rumen fill
- Cow cleanliness (udder, thigh and hips, legs)
- Signs of heat stress (> 70 respirations/minute)
- % cows ruminating at rest
- % of cows lying down and ruminating
- Cow 'comfort' and contentment (obviously hungry and unsettled)
- Flight zone (< 3 m, 3 to 5 m, > 5 m)
- Evidence of good or poor stock handling practices
- Herd numbers and structure
  - ➤ Milking cows
  - ➤ Dry cows
  - ➤ Heifers (weaning to calving)
  - ➤ Milk-fed calves
  - ➤ Other dairy stock (bulls, steers)

Feed supplies
- Enough fresh forage fed each day? Typical amount fed per milking cow in wet/dry season
- State of forage (improved v native v forage by-products, immature v mature)
- Sourcing fresh forage, grown v off farm
- Enough concentrates fed each day? Typical amount fed per cow
- Concentrates (formulated v mixed)
- What by-products are fed?

- If on farm mixing, specific feed additives (macro minerals, vitamins/minerals, rumen buffers)
- Use of shed effluent for forage production

Answers to simple questions
- How many cows did you milk yesterday?
- How much milk did you sell yesterday?
- How much milk did you use to feed your milk-fed calves yesterday?

These answers should allow you to calculate the average milk yield per milking cow:

- How much per kg of milk were you paid yesterday?
- If there is a milk grading scheme, what grade was your milk yesterday?
- What was the typical composition of your milk (fat, solids not fat, protein)?
- What was the typical quality of your milk (measured using somatic cell count, toal plate count or TPC, Methelyne blue reductase test or MBRT)?

Answers to more complex questions
- How aware are you of the importance of colostrum feeding to your newborn calves and what are your normal practices?

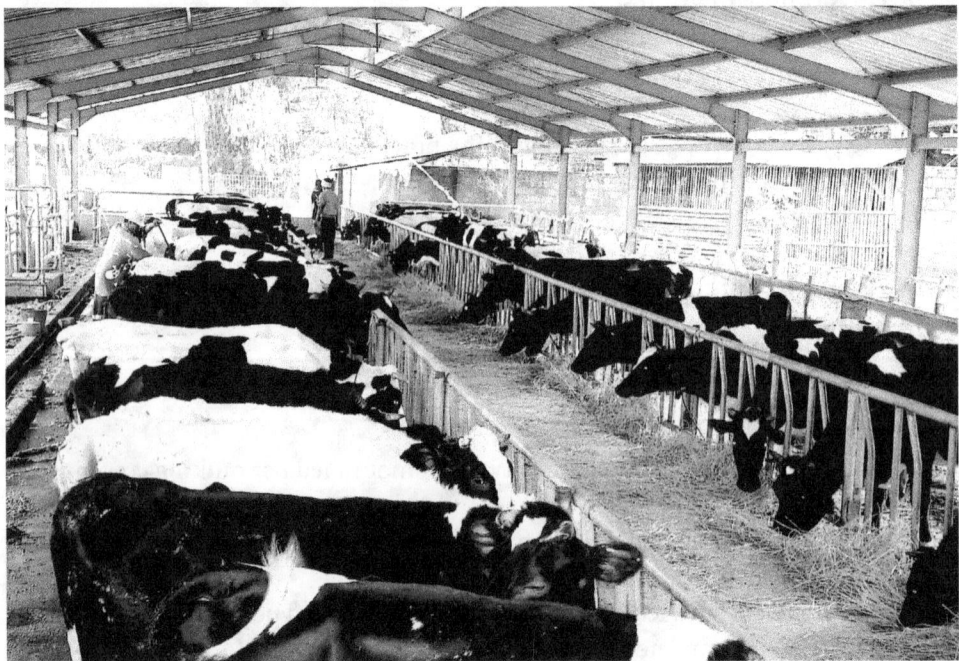

Figure 9.4: Cow colony incorporating many small holder farmers' animals.

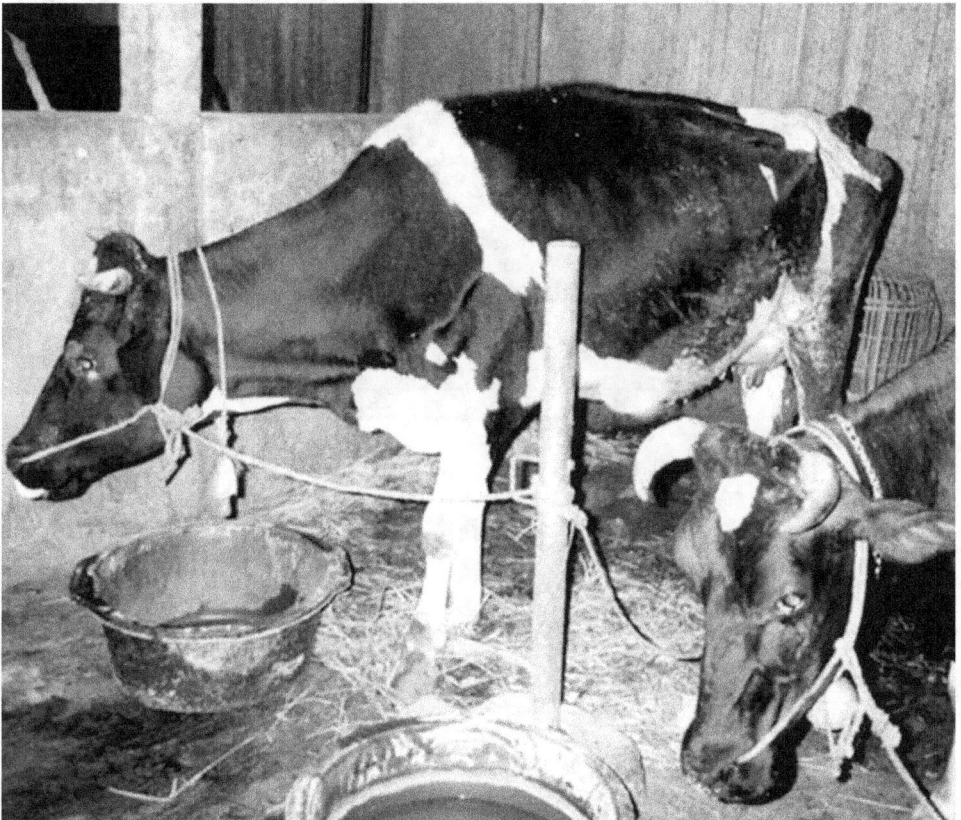

Figure 9.5: Cows continuously tethered in a darkened shed.

- Do you keep any farm records? If so, which ones?
- What financial/business records do you keep?
- Do you consider mastitis to be a problem?
- Do you consider cow lameness to be a problem?
- What is the typical peak yield of your cows in early lactation?
- What is the typical lactation length of your cows (< 250, 250–275, 275–300, > 300 days)?
- What are your typical number of days between calving to conception?
- What is your typical number of days between cows drying off and then calving?
- What is your typical age (number of months) of heifers when they first calve down?
- What is your typical percentage of calves that show signs of ill health during milk rearing?
- What is your typical percentage of calves that die during milk rearing?

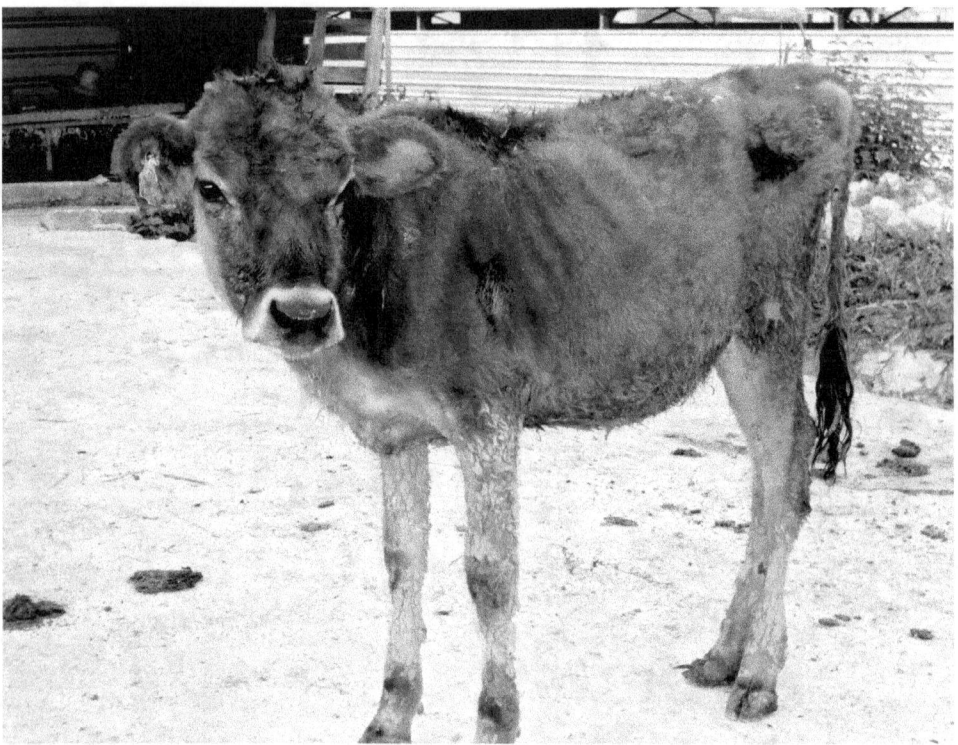

Figure 9.6: A very poorly reared Jersey dairy heifer.

- How many years have you been milking cows?
- Will you still be milking cows in a year's time or 5 years' time?
- Do your children want to follow you on the farm?
- Name three of your biggest problems on your farm. This can be any constraint at all, such as labour supplies, government/co-op or milk processor support and services, dry season forage supplies. Poor milk returns and high cost of production are universal problems for all small holder dairy farmers, so should not be included unless they are an obvious problem on this farm.

Figures 9.4, 9.5 and 9.6 illustrate cow welfare in SE Asia in different farm systems that can all be improved with better farm management practices.

10

A protocol for the welfare of stock on tropical small holder dairy farms

This chapter presents a protocol for the welfare of stock on tropical small holder dairy (SHD) farms.

The main points of this chapter

- A protocol is a series of Standard Operating Procedures that describe instructions for any activity or set of tasks undertaken on the farm. Stock, as well as people, perform better when all farm practices are undertaken in a routine manner.
- The protocol in this chapter is based on the 'five basic freedoms' of livestock. They are freedom from hunger, from thirst, discomfort or pain, fear and distress as well as the freedom to express normal behaviour. These form the basic elements of many national and international animal welfare protocols:
  1. Ensure animals are free from hunger and thirst through ready access to fresh water and a diet to maintain full health and vigour to produce healthy productive animals.
  2. Ensure animals are free from discomfort through provision of appropriate shelter and comfortable resting areas to protect animals against extreme climatic conditions and to provide them with a safe environment.
  3. Ensure animals are free from pain, injury and disease by prevention and, when sick, rapid diagnosis and treatment to ensure humane

actions, good sanitary conditions, prompt attention when required and, if necessary, humane destruction.

4. Ensure animals are free from fear and distress by ensuring conditions and treatment that avoids mental suffering and ensures safety of animals and people.

5. Ensure animals are free to express normal behaviour by providing adequate space, proper facilities and the company of other animals to preserve their gregarious and other favourable behavioural traits.

This chapter is the culmination of this manual in that it sets out a protocol for the welfare of stock on SHD farms in the tropics. A protocol is a list of instructions or guidelines on how best to do things to achieve success in the farming venture, which in this case is the dairy enterprise. Although the emphasis is on small holder farms, its principles are equally relevant for larger farms. The protocol is simply a collection of farm management activities called Standard Operating Procedures.

10.1   Standard Operating Procedures

A Standard Operating Procedure (SOP) is a formal term used to describe a set of instructions for any activity or set of tasks undertaken in the workplace. It should be described in sufficient detail that any non-skilled person could attempt to undertake it. Such SOPs can be developed to be the most suitable procedures to achieve the most desirable, or the best possible, outcome, in which case they become best management practices (BMP).

It is important to develop SOPs for major farm tasks because on large farms they are likely to be carried out by more than one farm worker. The benefits of SOPs include:

- They lead to consistency even when undertaken by different people.
- Stock perform better if routines do not change.
- People thrive on consistency – they know the instructions to follow on how to do a particular job and what the outcome should be.
- Training new staff is easier as there are carefully documented steps to achieve a specific outcome.
- As they are written down, any member of the farm staff can refresh their memory on how to perform the tasks.
- They can be referred to by managers to follow through any farm activity that did not give the desired outcome.
- They can even be used as legal documents in the case of formal disputes.

Generic SOPs can be developed for any set of tasks but the best ones are those developed in collaboration with the staff (workers and management) who are actually carrying them out, because they are the ones most familiar with the farm operations and the infrastructure, equipment and methods used on that particular farm.

A simple approach to developing an SOP is as follows:

- Prioritise the areas that would benefit from an SOP, namely, those that would most benefit from a series of clear written protocols.
- Select the most appropriate farm staff to oversee the development of the SOP, obviously those with overall responsibility for that task.
- Ensure that anyone likely to undertake this task is involved in its development.
- Make a list of processes, within the selected area.
- Identify the extent of what the SOP covers and what it does not.
- Give the SOP a specific name.
- Detail its scope within the farming system.
- Additional contents of SOPs can include:
  - ➤ Prominently list hazards that exist and precautions that should be taken.
  - ➤ Detail any safety equipment or protective clothing required.
  - ➤ List all equipment and supplies needed.
  - ➤ Detail, in sequence, the steps needed to be taken to achieve the desired outcome.

Once completed, a brief summary of the SOP can be placed in a convenient location, such as on a wall in the cowshed. The more detailed SOP should be located in the farm office, with a copy also in the staff quarters. This should be reviewed, say, every 12 months and updated to remain pertinent to the task.

10.2 Animal welfare protocols for dairy stock on tropical small holder farms

The guiding principle and objective of good dairy farming practice is that safe, quality milk should be produced from healthy animals using management practices that are sustainable from an animal welfare, social, economic and environmental perspective. Farmers then need to apply good practice in the following areas of their management:

- Animal health
- Milking hygiene
- Nutrition (feed and water)
- Animal welfare
- Environment
- Socioeconomic management.

To provide a framework to achieve these objectives, the Food and Agriculture Organisation (2011) published their *Guide to good dairy farming practice*. The essential elements of the animal welfare component of this guide were originally formulated by the International Dairy Federation (2008), based on Brambell's (1965) 'five basic freedoms' of livestock, that have been discussed in Section 8.1.1. Although the guide was written generically for farmers producing milk from any dairy species in any global environment, the animal welfare section provides a good protocol for SHD farmers in the tropics. In so doing, this protocol:

- Highlights relevant aspects that need to be proactively managed on farm.
- Identifies the desired outcomes in dealing with each aspect.
- Specifies good farming practices that address the critical hazards.
- Provides examples of control measures that should be implemented to achieve the objectives.
- Focuses on the desired outcomes rather than on specific prescriptive actions or processes.
- Concentrates on the practices rather than the principles of good animal welfare.

The recommendations for stock welfare protocols form the remainder of this chapter. These protocols do not include any actual numbers, such as minimum recommendations for the length of feeding spaces or the size of resting areas for dairy stock as these often vary with the type of production system (such as tethering v loose housing). They have been discussed fully in this book's earlier chapters and the senior author's previous tropical dairy farming manuals.

10.2.1 *Ensure animals are free from hunger and thirst,* through ready access to fresh water and a diet to maintain full health and vigour to produce healthy productive animals

Provide sufficient feed and water for all animals every day

Dairy livestock should be given sufficient feed, based on their physiological needs. Their requirements will vary according to their age, bodyweight, stage of lactation, production level, growth, pregnancy, activity and environment. Provide enough space around feeding and watering points to reduce bullying and ensure all livestock have sufficient access.

The quality (palatability and nutrient content) of the feed also needs to be considered, based on the animal's dietary requirements. Dietary supplements need to be considered if the ration is unable to meet the animal's nutrient requirements. Animals should be fed a balanced diet and have continual access to clean water.

Adjust farm stocking capacities and/or supplementary feeding to ensure adequate water, feed and fodder supply

Due consideration should be given to the number of animals, their physiological needs and the nutrient quality of feeds when determining farm stocking capacities. All animals should have access to sufficient water each day.

Protect animals from toxic plants and other harmful substances
Protect animals from access to toxic plants and contaminated areas such as farm dumps. Do not feed animals mouldy feeds. Store chemicals securely to avoid contamination of feeds, and observe withholding periods for any pasture or forage that undergoes chemical treatments.

Provide water supplies of good quality that are regularly checked and maintained
Animals should have free access to a clean fresh water supply. Regularly clean water troughs or drinkers and inspect them to ensure they are fully functional. The water supply should be adequate to meet peak requirements. Drinkers/water troughs should fill sufficiently quickly to avoid any animals in a group remaining thirsty. All reasonable steps should be taken to minimise the risks of the water supply freezing or overheating, as appropriate. Run-off from effluent and chemical treatments of pasture and forage crops should not enter stock water supplies.

10.2.2 *Ensure animals are free from discomfort,* through provision of appropriate shelter and comfortable resting areas to protect animals against extreme climatic conditions and to provide them with a safe environment

Design and construct buildings and handling facilities to be free of obstructions and hazards
Consideration should be given to the free flow of animals when designing and building animal housing and/or milking sheds. Avoid dead ends, and steep and slippery pathways. Ensure dairy buildings are safely wired and properly earthed.

Provide adequate space allowances and clean bedding
Avoid overcrowding of animals, even for short periods. Keep animal group sizes manageable and provide adequate feeding and watering space to reduce aggressive competitive behaviours.

Dairy cattle have strong herding instincts. Group animals by similar weight and size if possible. Manage herd introductions to reduce fighting, particularly between mature and intact males.

Provide housed animals with adequate space for resting on comfortable bedding and protected from hard surfaces such as concrete. These areas should be kept clean (e.g. by replacing the bedding frequently). Grazing areas are usually suitable for resting, provided that they are rotated frequently and have adequate drainage.

Protect animals from adverse weather conditions and the consequences thereof
As far as practicable, protect animals from adverse weather conditions and the consequences arising from such conditions. This includes stress factors such as

weather extremes, forage shortages, unseasonal changes and others causing cold or heat stress. Consider shade or alternative means of cooling such as misters and sprays. In cold conditions, shelter such as windbreaks and housing, and additional feed should be provided. Permanent shelters with lightning arresters may be warranted in some areas. Have plans to protect dairy animals against emergencies (for example back-up power supplies) and natural disasters (for example fire, drought, snow and flood). Include provision of high ground in case of flood, provide adequate firebreaks and have evacuation provisions.

Provide housed animals with adequate ventilation
All animal housing should be adequately ventilated allowing a sufficient supply of fresh air to remove humidity, allow heat dissipation and prevent build-up of gases such as carbon dioxide, ammonia or slurry gases.

Provide suitable flooring and safe footing in housing and animal traffic areas
Floors should be constructed to minimise slipping and bruising due to slippery or uneven floors. Excessively rough concrete or surfaces with sharp protrusions and stones can cause excessive wear or penetrations to the sole of the hoof, resulting in lameness. Unsuitable floors may inhibit mounting behaviours and lead to injuries. Protective floor coverings (e.g. rubber matting or other non-slip surfaces) can be used on walkways to reduce hoof abrasions that lead to secondary hoof infections and lameness.

Protect animals from injury and distress during loading and unloading and provide appropriate conditions for transport
Transport can pose risks to the welfare of dairy animals. Ensure the loading and unloading facilities are adequate and that water is available in lairage, if appropriate. Ensure the vehicle is suitably constructed to safely contain the animals, has good footing and adequate space allowances. If longer journeys have to be made, careful planning is required to ensure statutory welfare (feed, watering and resting) requirements are met.

10.2.3 *Ensure animals are free from pain, injury and disease* by prevention and, when sick, rapid diagnosis and treatment to ensure humane actions, good sanitary conditions, prompt attention when required and, if necessary, humane destruction

Have an effective herd health management program in place and inspect animals regularly
Animals should be regularly checked to detect injury and/or disease. Treatment and preventative herd health management programs should be in place.

Do not use procedures and processes that cause unnecessary pain
People carrying out veterinary related tasks should be able to demonstrate competency, especially for procedures that could cause suffering, for example, disbudding/dehorning, castration, etc. Adhere to national regulations with respect to these and other practices (such as hot branding, tail docking, teat amputations and so on). Good hygiene is essential for surgical-type procedures. Consider alternative animal husbandry practices if appropriate.

Follow appropriate birthing and weaning practices
Develop an appropriate birthing plan that considers such issues as choice of sire (for ease of birthing); safe birthing facilities and regular checking of animals to ensure prompt, experienced help is provided if required. Newborn animals should be fed colostrum within their first 12 to 24 h of life. Wean young dairy animals once they are consuming sufficient dry feed.

Have appropriate procedures for marketing young dairy animals
Calves should not be offered for sale until sufficiently hardy to be transported. Adequate bodyweight and dry navel are good indicators. Appropriate transport conditions stipulated in national welfare regulations or codes of practice should be followed.

Protect against lameness
Laneways, yards, milking stalls and housing should be constructed to minimise the incidence of lameness. Regular hoof care management practices should be implemented and the animals' diets adjusted to minimise lameness. Lameness should be investigated to determine underlying causes and treated appropriately. Allow animals to move at their own pace.

Milk lactating animals regularly
Establish a regular milking routine appropriate to the stage of lactation that does not overly stress the animals.

Avoid poor milking practices as they may injure animals
Poor milking practices can affect animal wellbeing and production. Milking equipment should be well maintained and regularly serviced.

When animals have to be killed on-farm, avoid unnecessary stress or pain
When it is necessary to kill sick or diseased animals, or those in pain, it should be done promptly and in such a manner as to avoid unnecessary pain and distress.

10.2.4 *Ensure animals are free from fear and distress* by ensuring conditions and treatment that avoid mental suffering and ensure the safety of animals and people

Consider animal behaviour when developing farm infrastructure and herd management routines

Good design of facilities that takes into account the natural behaviours of dairy animals can enhance the movement of animals on the farm. It will also benefit the stock handlers as the number of negative interactions will be reduced. Quiet, consistent handling practices using well-designed facilities promote better productivity and safety from reduced fear and stress.

Provide competent stock handling and husbandry skills and appropriate training

Good stock handling and husbandry skills are key factors in animal welfare. Without competent, diligent farm workers who take good care of animals in their charge, the cows' welfare will be compromised.

A competent operator should be able to:

- recognise whether or not the animals are in good health
- understand the significance of a change in the behaviour of the animals
- know when veterinary treatment is required
- implement a planned herd health management program, such as preventive treatments or vaccination programs when necessary
- implement appropriate animal feeding and grassland management programs
- recognise if the general environment (indoors or outdoors) is adequate to promote good health and welfare
- have management skills appropriate to the scale and technical requirements of the production system
- handle animals compassionately and in an appropriate manner
- anticipate potential problems and take the necessary preventive action.

Staff should be familiar with and comply with all relevant national regulations and key industry standards/assurance schemes relating to product quality/safety, etc. Staff should ensure records are maintained to demonstrate compliance with regulations or assurance schemes. People already involved in animal management/husbandry should keep themselves updated on technological developments that can prevent or correct welfare problems.

Use facilities and equipment that are suitable for stock handling

Ensure the facilities and equipment used to handle the animals are appropriate for the purpose, well designed and maintained. This can avoid injury to both people and the animals. Careful use of equipment can reduce fear in animals and make

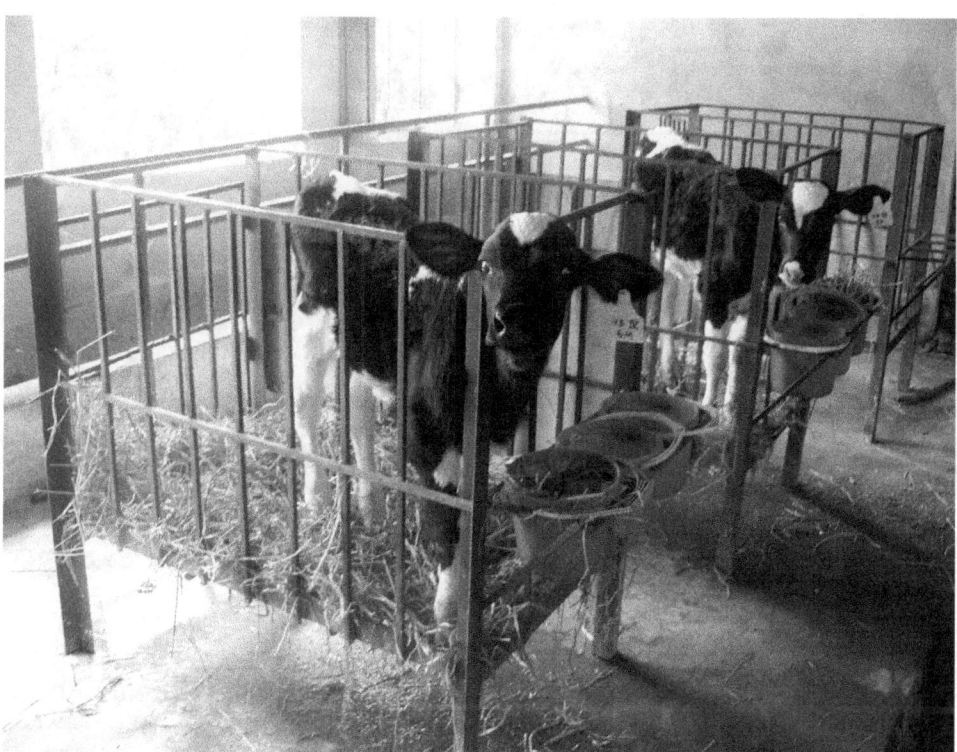

Figure 10.1: Milk-fed calves should be kept clean and dry with adequate water as well as dry feed and milk. They do not feel isolated because they can easily see each other.

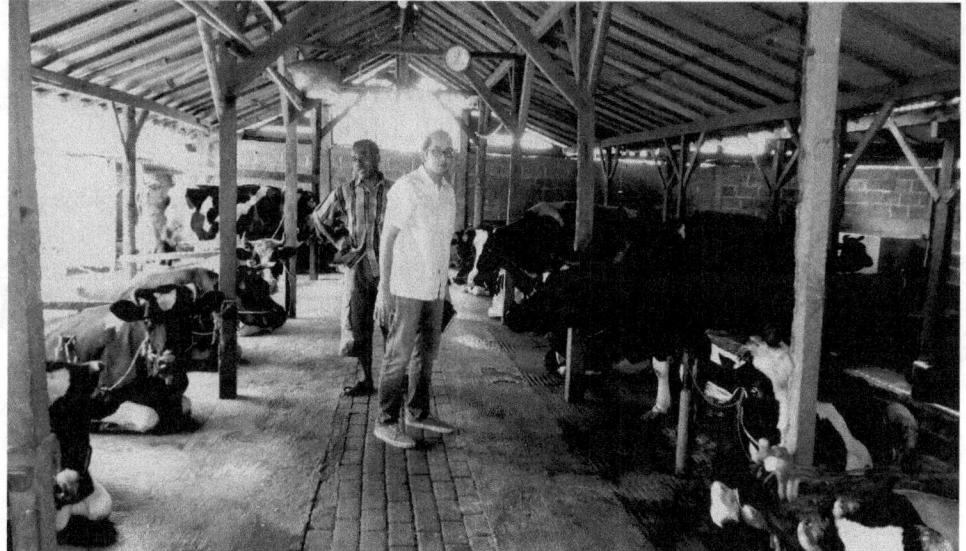

Figure 10.2: A typical tropical small holder dairy farm with a low roofed and poorly ventilated shed, permanently tethered stock and no rubber mats.

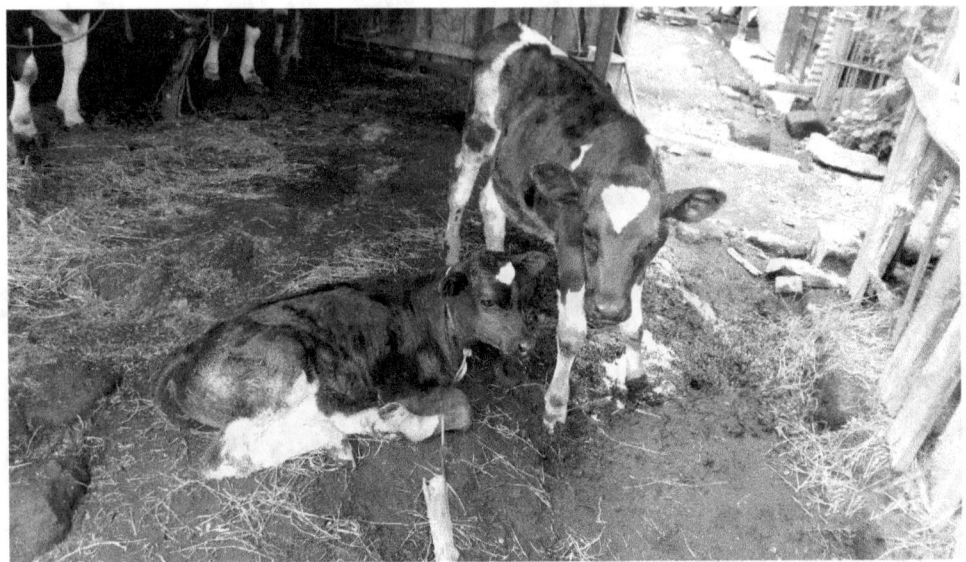

Figure 10.3: These calves have no comfortable place to lie on.

them easier and safer to handle. Monitor the animals' behaviour to identify aspects of the facilities or equipment that may provoke fear or be causing discomfort.

10.2.5 *Ensure animals are free to express normal behaviour* by providing adequate space, proper facilities and the company of other animals to preserve their gregarious and other favourable behavioural traits

Have herd management and husbandry procedures that do not unnecessarily compromise the animals' resting and social behaviours

Dairy stock are gregarious animals (Figure 10.1). Use herd management and husbandry procedures that do not unnecessarily compromise their natural behaviours, such as herding, feeding, reproductive and resting behaviours. This also means sufficient space should be provided for these activities (Figures 10.2 and 10.3). During the daily inspection(s) of animals, check for any abnormal behaviour. Ensure each animal has adequate space to feed appropriately and actually is feeding. Failure to feed may be an early indication of illness in an animal. Mature and intact males should be managed and handled in a manner that promotes good temperament and prevents aggression towards other stock and staff.

11

Conclusions

This chapter concludes the manual with some final overviews, such as the role of a demonstration or model farm in promoting good animal welfare practices to reach the widest audience possible.

The main points of this chapter

- Closer attention needs to be given to the economics of current small holder dairy (SHD) systems. Sourcing high yielding dairy cows, but providing the feeding and management that only utilises a small proportion of their potential, is just not sustainable in the long run.
- Local milking cows will often perform similarly to the imported animal under traditional levels of herd management, they are two to three times cheaper to purchase and are likely to be more resilient to poor welfare practices.
- To ensure sustainability, the current production systems need to evolve into more resource efficient ones, and this includes providing closer attention to cow comfort and hence cow welfare. Such systems will require more skilled farmers and better-trained support staff, so there needs to be greater emphasis given to farmer training and capacity building programs.
- No matter how much the animal welfare and extreme animal liberation lobby groups speak out against the farming of cattle for milk and meat, it is certain that humans will never cease cattle farming. Commercial and

nationalistic interests will continue to facilitate the global distribution of dairy and beef cattle from regions approaching or exceeding self-sufficiency to other regions where demands for milk and meat far exceed supplies.

- High performing genotypes require excellent farm management to help them achieve their potential. Under the more traditional farm management that exists in many tropical SHD systems, such animals will often perform less well than the local stock.
- Recent studies in Bangladesh suggest that Jersey crossbreds may be more suitable and productive than Friesian crossbreds on traditionally managed SHD farms.
- Farmers are experiential learners. They learn more by doing something themselves (and being able to monitor its impact) than by the more traditional learning programs of classroom tuition and short 'hands on' practical sessions. Model farms provide them with a practically based learning environment.
- The model farm should then be established to provide farmers and service providers with an overview of the cause and effect of modifications in farm practices. This is ideally suited to demonstrate the beneficial impacts of improved animal welfare.
- This chapter lists a series of improved management practices that can be demonstrated on a model farm.
- Competent, welfare-minded dairy farmers are those who extend their farming skills to cover cow psychology as well as cow production technology and farm business management. In essence, they should be able to put themselves 'inside the cow's skin' to develop the ability to 'think like a cow'.
- Happy cows make happy farmers.

11.1 Considering current production constraints on tropical dairy farms

This manual covers a wide range of topics primarily related to ensuring the sustainability of dairy production systems in tropical developing countries. Clearly, to achieve this aim, closer attention needs to be given to the economics of current systems. Sourcing high yielding dairy cows, but providing the feeding and management that only utilises a small proportion of their potential is just not sustainable in the long run. It is also a contributory factor to their suboptimal animal welfare. This is because such animals are more susceptible to the traumas of heat stress, poor housing conditions and all too often, subsistence feeding management. Currently the majority of these farms are only operating at a small fraction of their potential economic efficiency.

However, this observation must be viewed from the perspective that the SE Asian countries currently importing large numbers of dairy heifers from Western countries are unlikely ever to be able to greatly increase their national dairy cow populations through natural multiplication from within their own dairy herds. The local farmers suffer from poor reproductive performance (such as high ages at first calving and lengthy calving intervals) and high stock mortalities (particularly young replacement heifers). The major avenue to increase national herd sizes will have to be through continuing livestock importations.

No matter how much the animal welfare and extreme animal liberation lobby groups speak out against the farming of cattle for milk and meat, certainly humans will never cease cattle farming. Commercial and nationalistic interests will continue to facilitate the global distribution of dairy and beef cattle from regions approaching or exceeding self-sufficiency to other regions where demands for milk and meat far exceed supplies. This means that the animal welfare issues discussed in this book will always be there.

Producing more milk will then require purchasing more stock that will require lengthy periods of adaptation. These importing countries seem to prefer importing in-calf heifers rather than unbred, virgin heifers. However, even though they can purchase 'two high genetic animals for the price of one' (namely the pregnant heifer and her foetus), the heifers only have a few months to adapt to the local management conditions before she is expected to calve down then be able to conceive for her second calving. At least many of these heifers are now being transported by plane, which removes much of the transport stress suffered by heifers spending many weeks on ships. However, importing unbred heifers provides a much greater adaptation period before they are expected to produce milk then get back into calf again.

Two observations made by the senior author are pertinent in this discussion. First, in a herd of imported unbred heifers, all of which were cycling before air transportation, only 50% were still cycling, presumably due to the stresses of trying to adapt to their post-arrival feeding and herd management as well as their new climatic environment. The second observation was made at a farmer meeting in which he was told that 20 to 30% of the imported pregnant heifers suffered lactation anoestrus for so long post-calving that they were sent off to the local abattoir. One enterprising farmer identified these cows and purchased them before slaughter, provided them with good feeding, housing and welfare practices after which they all cycled and eventually conceived. Therefore, one must conclude that the reproductive endocrine responses in these cows due to their poor adaptation to suboptimal post-arrival management are likely to be more costly than those associated with milk synthesis in the udder.

With the costs of farm inputs destined to rise regularly, higher levels of cow and herd performance are necessary to ensure a reasonable profit margin for these farmers. It is just not good business sense to purchase such imported stock, say for US$2500 to 3000 each, then only feed and manage them to produce on average 10 to 12 L/cow/day of milk. Furthermore, the reproductive inefficiencies mentioned above will make it even less worthwhile. This is highlighted by the fact that up to 20% of progeny die during milk rearing and the surviving heifers frequently don't have their first calf until 30 to 36 months of age followed by a calving interval of 18 months. Local milking cows will often perform similarly to the imported animal under traditional levels of herd management, but are two to three times cheaper to purchase and likely to be more resilient to the existing poor welfare practices.

As standards of living improve, the cost of labour (both on farm and employed off farm labour) will rise. There is increasing competition, and therefore reduced availability, from both humans and other livestock sectors within each country, for the high quality feeds required to produce local milk. In addition, the costs of any imported dairy inputs, such as veterinary drugs and farm machinery, will only increase in the future. On the income side, the global markets will always place constraints on the maximum unit returns farmers can receive for their milk sales, as it is often cheaper to import the ingredients for processed dairy products. Therefore, future income and profit streams must come from increases in farm outputs of raw milk. To ensure sustainability, the current production systems need to evolve into more resource efficient ones. This includes providing closer attention to cow comfort and welfare. Such systems will require more skilled farmers and better-trained support staff which means there needs to be more emphasis given to farmer training and capacity building programs.

High levels of heat and humidity stress, inadequate levels of moderate quality feeds and less than ideal herd management practices, place enormous constraints on imported dairy animals. Future increasing concerns about the public accountability of animal welfare from exporting countries should (and eventually will) add another layer of concern to the future prospects for these countries to achieve their targeted levels of national self-sufficiency in dairy products.

Many of the SE Asian dairy industries have recently established large-scale dairy feedlots to provide more milk and so reduce imports of dairy products. However, these countries all have government-driven development policies for small or medium-sized farms to continue to supply the bulk of locally produced milk. This means existing farms will need to be better managed. Increased resources will also be required but these must be looked upon as future investments, not costs, in current dairy systems. Given better farm management and strategic investments, the increased levels of milk produced on such farms should provide sufficient profits – incentives to upgrading current farm management practices.

Frequently the text in this book has emphasised the impact of poor cattle welfare on animal performance and on the resultant farm profitability and potential sustainability. It is the obligation of all stakeholders in cattle farming to work steadfastly towards reducing stresses (psychological as well as physiological) on cattle as they have to cope with the current and improved production systems. Farmers, service providers, trainers and government/private bureaucrats are all stakeholders in cattle farming. Not only should they all become more familiar with key aspects of meat and milk production technology and farm business management, but the increasing public accountability of farmers towards the welfare of their stock should provide the incentive for them to also become more aware of the psychological needs of the stock under their control.

11.2   The genotypes of dairy stock imported onto tropical dairy farms

The intense genetic improvement programs for dairy stock being undertaken in the developed dairy industries of Australasia, North America and Europe will lead to higher genetic merit cows in the developing countries through continuing importations, such as in tropical Asia, Africa and Latin America. Such selection programs are leading to reductions in the genetic diversity of the world's dairy cow population. Such losses in genetic variability increase disease susceptibility in high producing genetic lines. For example, Phillips (2002) partly attributed the recent outbreak of 'mad cow disease' in the UK to the increased susceptibility to the disease due to the lack of genetic diversity in the country's population of Friesian dairy cows. This was a result of intense selection for high cow performance.

The more specialised a domestic animal becomes, the more specialised an environment it will require. For example, Friesians require better environmental support than a beef cow, that could survive under wild conditions. Friesian cows would greatly suffer in the wild with their huge udders, while their calves are weaker and take longer to walk unassisted compared to beef breed calves.

Selection for increased milk production and cow performance has continued for more than a century in Europe. It has produced dramatic results with cows producing more than 50 L/day of milk under optimal feeding and herd management. Dairy selection programs have also been undertaken in tropical regions utilising the tropical adaptation genes of Zebu (*Bos indicus*) stock. The resultant progeny have been nowhere near as productive as their temperate counterparts because of environmental and genetic constraints. The more recent importations of dairy stock to tropical developing countries have almost entirely been based on Friesians. This has been primarily due to the often mistaken belief that such stock would always be the most productive in their new environment.

Even within the temperate dairy gene pool, there are breeds that exhibit a greater degree of tropical adaptation than do Friesians, such as Jersey, Brown Swiss and Red Danish. In addition, there are synthetic dairy breeds bred specifically for tropical conditions that – although in short supply – could be the centre of a breed multiplication scheme within the host country. Such breeds include the Australian Friesian Sahiwal, Australian Milking Zebu, the Brazilian Girolando and purebred Sahiwal.

High performing genotypes require excellent farm management to help them achieve their potential. Under the more traditional farm management that exists in many tropical SHD systems, such animals will often perform poorly compared with the local stock. This is primarily because of their propensity to preferentially utilise their body reserves to produce milk during early lactation. Without sufficient nutrient intakes, they will lose weight and upset the hormonal balances to allow them to regain their normal oestrus cycle for many months following calving. Reduced reproductive performance of high grade Friesians is an all too common feature of traditional feeding and herd management on tropical SHD farms. As already mentioned, the inability to get back in calf within several months due to lactation anoestrus can represent up to 20 or 30% of imported dairy stock being culled and slaughtered after just one lactation (Moran 2012a).

The following Table 11.1 presents recent data derived from SHD farms in Bangladesh (Milk Vita 2013), relating to the genetic improvement of the local dairy animal, known as the Pabna Milking Cow (PMC) through cross breeding with established improved dairy breeds. The Sahiwal crossbreds were either Sahiwal x PMC or Sahiwal x (PMC x Friesian), the Friesian crossbreds were either Friesian x PMC or Friesian x (PMC x Sahiwal) while the Jerseys crossbreds were either Jersey x PMC or Jersey x (PMC x Sahiwal).

Compared to the Friesian crossbreds, the Jersey crossbreds were 3.2 kg lighter at birth but had a 12-day longer lactation length, produced an extra 131 kg milk

Table 11.1. Performance of three breed types in Bangladesh.

	Sahiwal	Friesian	Jersey
Birthweight (kg)	26.3	27.2	24.0
Lactation length (days)	282	290	302
Lactation yield (kg)	1735	2893	3024
Average milk yield (kg/d)	6.2	10.0	10.0
Fat%	4.4	4.1	4.9
Solids Not Fat (SNF) %	8.0	8.0	8.1
Age at first service (months)	29.8	27.1	25.0
Services per conception	1.3	1.7	1.2
Days to first post partum heat	137	149	98
Calving interval (days)	419	430	382

over their entire lactation and had an 0.8% higher fat% and 0.1% more Solids Not Fat contents. In addition, they were 2.1 months younger at first service, required 51 days less to first post partum heat, and 0.5 less services per conception and subsequently had a 48-day shorter calving interval. Western data usually show Jerseys producing less milk per day than Friesians but these data showed identical daily milk yields (10.0 kg/cow/day). The poorer performance of the Sahiwals compared to the Friesian crossbreds is also apparent from these data, although the Sahiwals required fewer services per conception, had fewer days to first post partum heat and shorter calving intervals than the Friesians. Clearly, under traditional management in a hot and humid environment where cows were only producing 10 kg/cow/d on average, Jersey crossbreds performed better than Friesian crossbreds.

No matter what genotype is favoured for dairy development programs, farm management practices almost always can be rectified to better achieve their productive potential (Figures 11.1 and 11.2). Not only do these improvements need to be directed towards providing better cow comfort and nutrient status, a more concerted effort in addressing all aspects of cow welfare will almost always reap benefits (Figure 11.3).

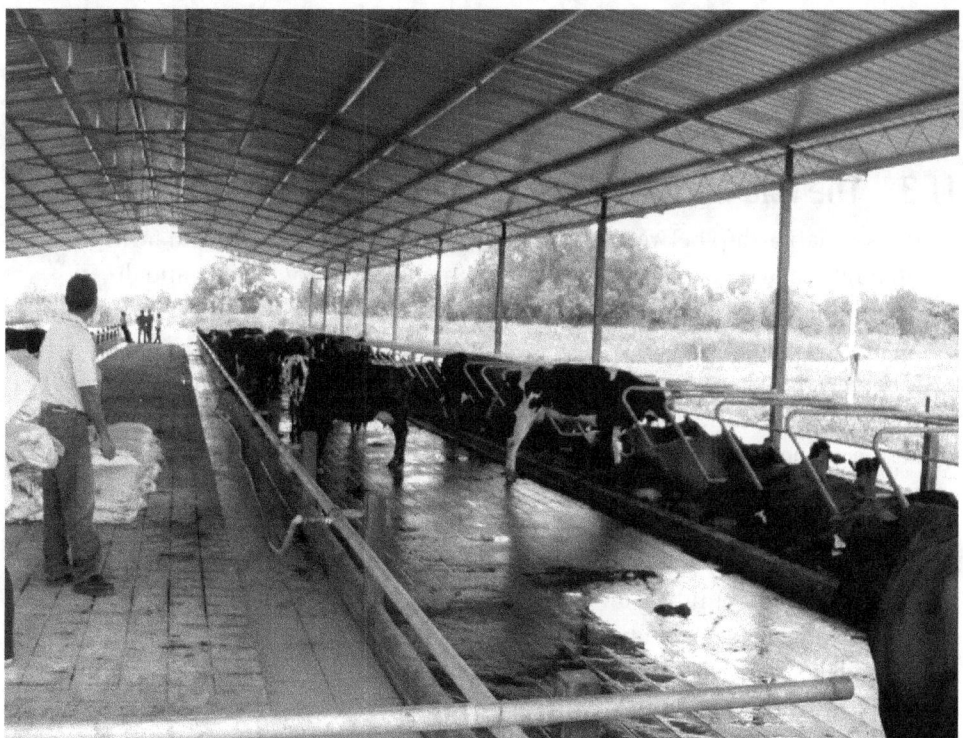

Figure 11.1: A well-designed and managed free stall shed in the tropics.

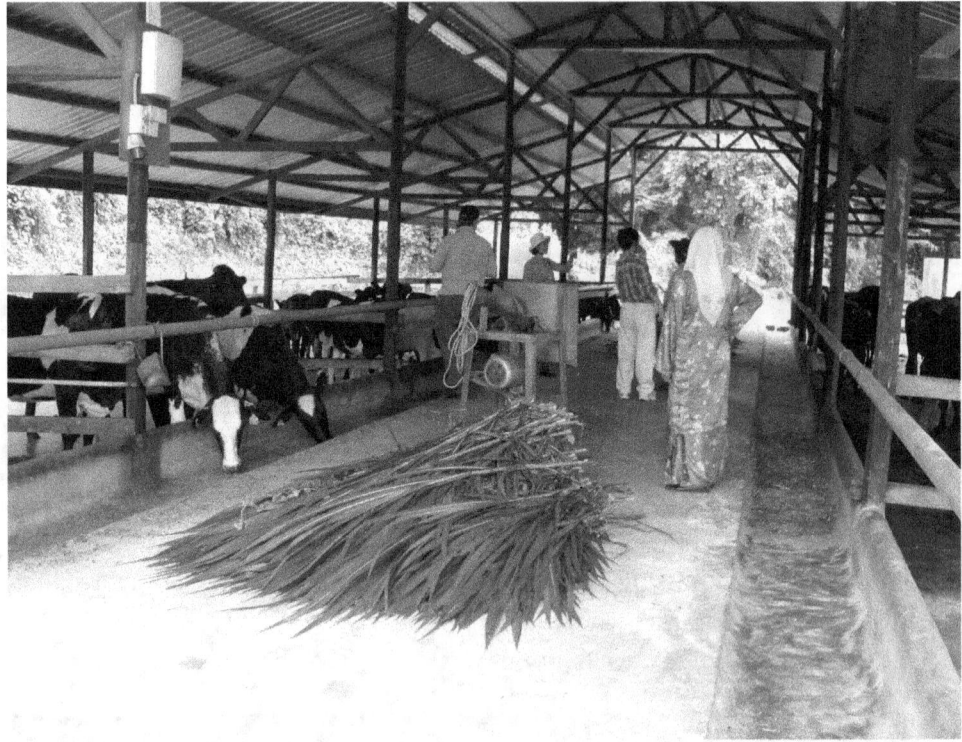

Figure 11.2: A well-managed small holder dairy shed in the tropics.

11.3 The role for model farms

The close relationship between animal welfare, cow performance and farm profitability on SHD farms has been highlighted throughout this manual. Similarly, the text has laid emphasis on the general lack of awareness of this association by poorly resourced tropical farmers. Farmer-orientated capacity building programs are then a high priority to rectify this deficiency.

Changes in a single farm practice can have a diversity of outcomes. Unlike researchers who use traditional approaches to scientific logic in a research environment, to try and hold all other variables constant when assessing the impact of one particular variable, farmers live in the 'real world of commercial agriculture' where any single variable can rarely be held constant on farm. Therefore, capacity building for poorly resourced and skilled farmers should ideally be undertaken on a farm.

A model or demonstration farm highlights the dynamic nature of farming as it can expose farmers to practical innovations and new ideas. There are various ways in which such innovations can be introduced to a group of farmers, but the

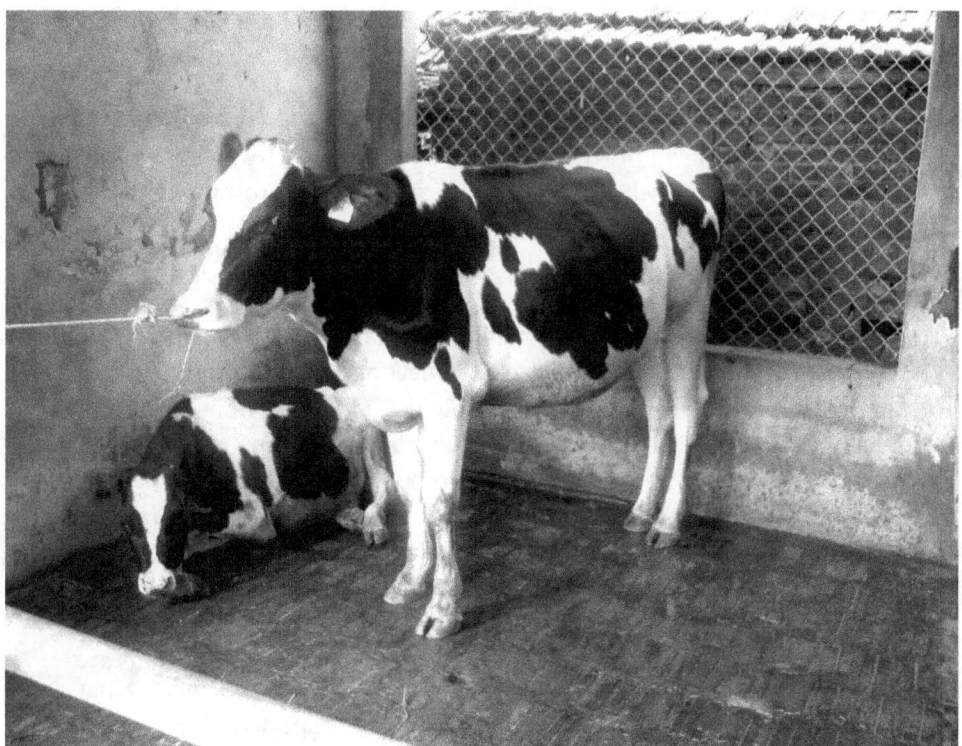

Figure 11.3: A 24-month-old pregnant dairy heifer, the result of good feeding, management and welfare.

important objective is for these farmers to understand how it impacts on 'the bottom line', that is the herd performance and farm profitability. In addition, animal welfare is a very complex part of farm management that unlike, say, feeding a better quality ration to milking cows to increase milk yields, is likely to impact on many aspects of herd performance when practice changes are made. In addition, animal welfare is directed to satisfy or improve the animals' coping mechanisms, with the success or otherwise being made apparent through a variety of performance parameters (as discussed in Chapter 8.2).

Farmers are experiential learners in that they learn more by doing something themselves (and being able to monitor its impact) rather than by the more traditional learning programs of classroom tuition and short 'hands on' practical sessions. However, classroom sessions are important because they provide the opportunity to explain the theories behind such practices, which are an integral component of any learning process. Better comprehension of 'why things happen' will improve the understanding of 'how to make things happen', because all too frequently 'things do not go according to plan' because of various unknown and/or unexpected consequences of farmers' actions.

Since farmers learn more by watching and then doing, they need to be provided with every opportunity to watch. This can be provided on the farms of collaborating farmers, or better still, on a model farm. The latter is more desirable because there is more control over farm activities and it is easier to monitor the impacts of changes in farm practices. Using selected farmers who agree to allow their farms to be more closely monitored will provide a control situation so farmers can more easily see and understand the impact of any direct changes in herd performance and farm profitability as a result of such improved management practices.

The model farm should then be established to provide farmers and service providers with an overview of the cause and effect of modifications in farm practices. This is ideally suited to demonstrate the impacts of improved animal welfare. For example, the many benefits rising from the construction of a more 'cow friendly' shed can be demonstrated by comparing herd performance with that of an existing more traditional shed construction. As SHD farmers in many countries routinely travel twice each day to deliver their milk to the milk collection centre, establishing a model farm in close proximity to the collection centre, should encourage them to frequently visit it to monitor progress in any demonstration trial. Offering regular field days, at which the latest results are discussed, would further help in their dissemination. Although such a model farm may be the initiative of the public service providers, if well-managed and effective, it is likely to create interest within the private sector which could then be levered to provide additional resources for its operation.

11.3.1 Modus operandi of a model farm

Such a farm requires careful planning, preparation and construction to ensure it has a sustainable future as a farmer extension tool. The following is a list of some of the prerequisites:

- The farm should be located in established or soon to be established dairying regions, close to other commercial dairy enterprises.
- It should be of a commercial size and relevant to dairy farming within the next 5 to 10 years, say, between 10 and 20 milking cows and associated young stock. If it is too large, small holder farmers will have difficulty relating to it and so adopting any improved management practices. The size of the forage production area should be such as to provide fresh forage for, say, 8 to 10 milking cows per ha forage per year. This may or may not include home-grown forages conserved as silage.
- The facilities should be constructed of materials that are readily available and likely to be used by local dairy farmers.

- It should be stocked with imported cows and young stock, assuming these will become the future benchmark of developing dairy industries.
- The farm should be managed by an experienced SHD farmer with a proven track record of innovative dairy farming.
- The day-to-day management would be the responsibility of the manager. However, the manager should be supported by an advisory group of experienced dairy specialists. These should represent a range of agencies, from the investors, to large-scale milk processors, dairy cooperatives and government (and maybe expatriate) dairy advisers and maybe educational institutes. This group would meet several times each year to monitor progress in the farm's economic performance as well as its role as an extension tool.
- The farm must be operated as a commercial business with additional resources available to develop effective extension activities, such as regular visits from local dairy farmers and other dairy stakeholders.
- The milk produced should be sold through the normal market outlets, either through a milk collection centre or direct to an established milk processor. Consideration could be given at a later date to value add some of the milk.
- The initial finances to purchase (or rent) the land and construct the facilities could be sourced from agribusiness, and maybe even government or other dairy industry stakeholders. The stakeholders will then be invited to become involved in the overall management of the farm.
- As well as documenting cow and farm performance, all data on cash inputs and outputs should be collated and regularly summarised to form an integral part of the extension message.
- There should be regular meetings (small groups of farmers visiting) and an annual regional forum to demonstrate and extend the correct farm management practices.

11.3.2   Examples of improved management practices

The following list shows some of the improved management practices, many of which will lead to better animal welfare, that could be demonstrated on a model farm:

Sheds and facilities
Loose housing rather than tie stalls
Free stalls rather than open lounging
Compost barn as an open lounging system
Rubber mats in the free stalls
Outside sand yard for resting at night
Good slope on floor to aid cleaning

Flood wash system to clean floor
Cow shed design: adequate height and open sides
Cattle crush and yards for ease of handling stock
Mating yard, if using bulls not AI
Young stock rearing area not directly adjacent to adult cow area
Individual pens or cages for milk rearing calves
Effluent dam to minimise nitrogen losses through volatilisation
Pump and pipes to distribute liquid effluent onto forage production area
Mechanical milking, not hand milking, probably with bucket milkers
Hot water to clean milk handling and milk feeding equipment
Separate area in which cows can give birth
Hospital or isolation pen for sick stock
Vermin-free and insect-proof storage area for feeds
Refrigerator and lockable cabinet for drug storage
Fans and maybe even sprinklers for heat stress management
Plant trees and grass around sheds
Area for staff to relax when not working
Office area for keeping and storing farm records

Feed and forage management
Routine use of inorganic fertilisers on grass production area
Short harvest interval for Napier grass (30 days not 60 days)
Consider routine wilting of freshly harvested forage to improve appetite and hence increase productivity
Consider making silage out of excess wet season forage to feed back to stock in dry season
If using raw ingredients for concentrate formulations, a separate area for mixing them on the floor
Ensure farms can source adequate supplies of quality forages to make up for any shortfalls in home-grown forages
Ensure farms can source adequate supplies of quality ingredients for supplementing forages
Provision of continuous supplies of fresh clean drinking water
Harvesting and feeding adequate quantities of quality green forages (say 40 kg/cow/d) to milking herd
Use mechanical chopper for processing forages
Consider ribbon mixer or small total mixed ration (TMR) wagon to mix all the feed ingredients
Consider routine analyses of nutritive value of all feed inputs
Formulate rations based on minimum costs of feed energy and protein within each feed type

Feed scales for weighing feeds
Chest girth tape for assessing stock live weights
Picture guides to routinely monitor body condition

Herd management practices
Feed colostrum to calves immediately following birth
Consider calf milk replacer as cheaper alternative to whole milk
Ensure calves are fed high protein concentrate formulations, not the same as for
    milking cows
Develop regular vaccination for young stock (*Clostridium*) as well as adult stock
Routinely monitor respiration rates to decide on heat stress alleviation procedures
Learn to identify early symptoms of ill health in calves, heifers and adult cows
Develop animal health protocols for milk-fed calves with local veterinarian
Develop animal health protocols for weaned heifers and adult cows with local
    veterinarian
Follow recommended Best Management Practices (BMP) for all aspects of herd
    management such as feeding, breeding, rearing young stock, milk harvesting,
    animal health and stock welfare
Do not use calves for milk letdown before milking
Only wash teats (not entire udder) when preparing cows for milking
Ensure cows stand for 30 min following milking
If using mechanical milking, change milk liners after every 2500 milkings
Routinely use pictorial standards (as in Chapter 6) to monitor various measures of
    stock welfare
Encourage staff to be involved in monitoring stock health and performance during
    their daily work routines, and writing observations down on a whiteboard
Collect sufficient production and financial data to routinely monitor the Key
    Performance Indicators discussed in Chapter 9.

11.4   In summary

In spite of several decades of dairy farming in the tropical developing countries of
SE Asia, the productivity of SHD farming has remained relatively low due in part
to the lack of appropriate dairy research and application. Small farmers, due to
their socioeconomic and agro-economic conditions being greatly different to those
in developed countries, cannot readily adopt the science and technology available
in developed countries. Even the most appropriate technology is rarely transferred
to small holders *en masse* due to a lack of effective support services (Moran 2014).
There needs to be large-scale institutional support to facilitate dairy industry
growth through mechanisms such as providers of farmer credit, farmer training
centres, well-equipped milk collection centres, processing and marketing facilities,

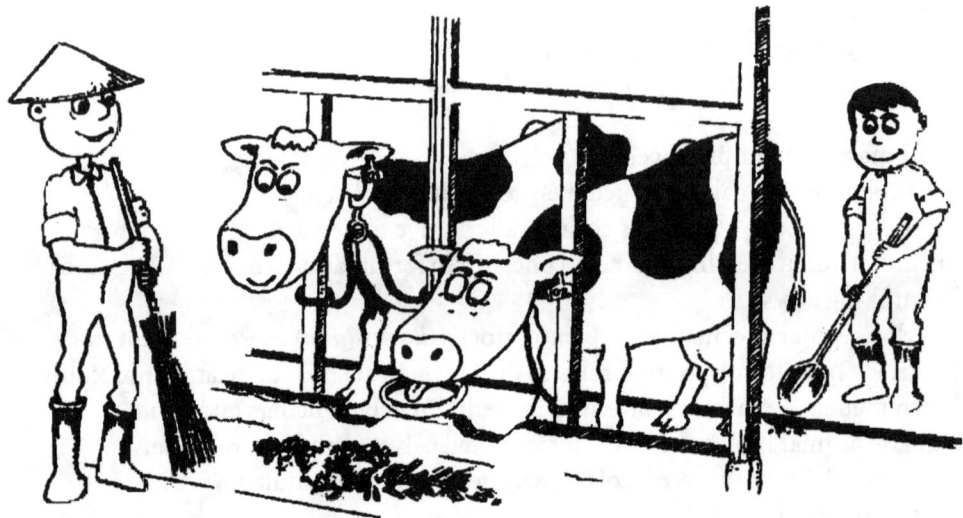

Figure 11.4: Happy cows on a well-managed small holder farm.

farmer cooperatives or groups and appropriate research and extension infrastructures and methodologies. School milk programs have been successful in encouraging the development of SHD farming by promoting milk drinking to improve health among children, particularly in rural areas. It is then essential for any production technology being transferred to these farmers to be relevant to

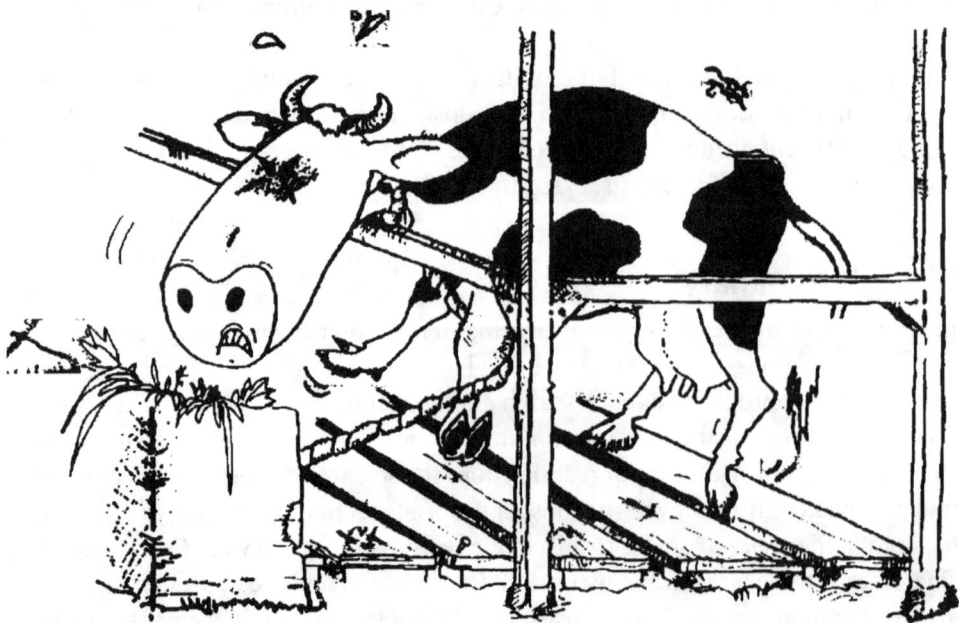

Figure 11.5: An unhappy cow on a poorly managed small holder farm.

their needs as well as being economically and practically feasible, given their local support networks of dairy cooperatives, advisers (government and agribusiness), creditors and milk handling and processing infrastructures. Production technology skills should automatically lead to animal welfare skills.

Good dairy cattle husbandry includes the provision of appropriate resources of feed and shelter, effective management and sympathetic stockpersonship. These include:

- Physical resources necessary to ensure proper feeding, housing and hygiene
  - ➤ Well-constructed, properly replenished feed stores
  - ➤ Accommodation that is hygienic, physically and thermally comfortable and unlikely to cause injury
  - ➤ Facilities for routine preventative medicine and the care of individual sick animals.
- Strategic management designed to address the physiological, health and behavioural needs of the animals
  - ➤ Feeding, production, health and welfare plans devised and implemented with professional advice as appropriate to the needs of the system and the individual animals
  - ➤ Comprehensive records relating to feeding, production, health and welfare.
- Competent stockpersonship, sympathetic to the day-to-day needs of the stock
  - ➤ A skilled empathetic approach to animal handling
  - ➤ Early recognition and attention to any signs of disease or injury
  - ➤ Work practices that encourage competent and caring stock handlers and which give them the time to develop empathy with the animals in their care.Competent, welfare-minded dairy farmers are those who extend their farming skills to cover cow psychology as well as cow production technology and farm business management. In essence, a farmer should be able to put themselves 'inside the cow's skin' to develop the ability to 'think like a cow'.

The term 'happy cow' is becoming more commonly used in dairy circles, particularly in Asian developing countries. In fact 'Happy cows, happy farmers' became a theme song at a recent dairy farmer meeting in Vietnam. The Figure 11.4 and 11.5 cartoons also promote the message that well-managed small holder farms produce happy cows.

Appendices

Appendix 1 Temperature Humidity Index

The following table presents the Temperature Humidity Index, calculated from temperature (in °Fahrenheit or Centigrade) and relative humidity (%), highlighting its potential effects on cow heat stress and hence performance.

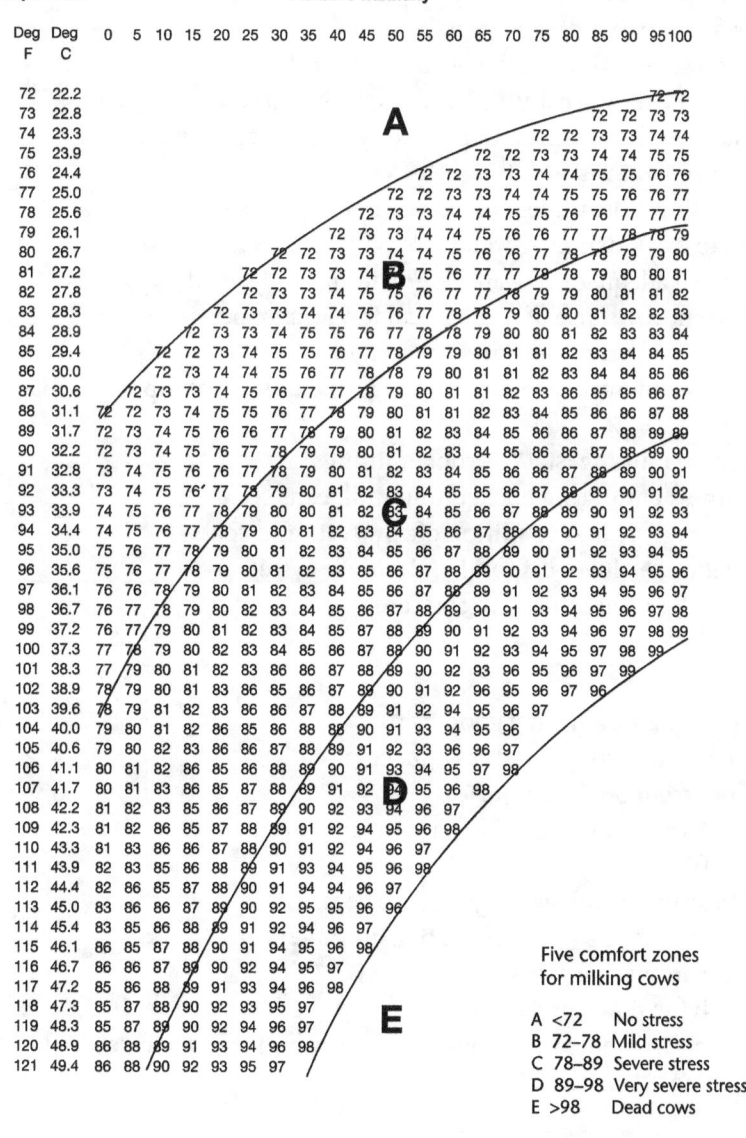

Five comfort zones for milking cows

A <72 No stress
B 72–78 Mild stress
C 78–89 Severe stress
D 89–98 Very severe stress
E >98 Dead cows

Appendix 2   Checklist to assess current farm management and herd welfare

These observations and answered questions can help assess the management and welfare of the stock and the performance and likely profitability of any farm.

Shed and facilities

- Roof height and natural ventilation
- Temperature and humidity inside shed
- Shed floor and cow lying area (cement, mats)
- Mats, enough for all cows, thin v thick
- Other forms of bedding material
- Stalls; tie stalls v free stalls v open lot
- General stocking density and space for cows to rest
- Adequacy and cleanliness of pens for young stock (heifers, milk-fed calves)
- Area for outside resting at night
- Adequacy and cleanliness of feed troughs and water containers
- Access to clean drinking water, not only as slurry feeding
- Source and adequacy of water for drinking and cleaning
- If sufficient cows, use of mechanical forage chopper
- Room for feed processing and preparation
- Adequacy and hygiene of milking area, including teat dipping and access to hot water
- If machine milking, state of rubber linings
- Cleanliness of milking buckets and milk cans
- General hygiene and condition of cow teats and coats
- Adequacy of effluent disposal and storage system
- Adequacy of office and farm staff area

Stock

- General condition (thin v good v fat)
- Obvious health issues, such as lameness
- Freedom from obvious injuries
- Is mastitis an issue? If so, what are the management procedures?
- Rumen fill
- Cow cleanliness (udder, thigh & hips, legs)
- Signs of heat stress (> 70 respirations/minute)
- % cows ruminating at rest
- % cows lying down and ruminating
- Cow 'comfort' and contentment (obviously hungry and unsettled)
- Flight zone (< 3 m, 3 to 5 m, > 5 m)

- Evidence of good or poor stock handling practices
- Herd numbers and structure
  - Milking cows
  - Dry cows
  - Heifers (weaning to calving)
  - Milk-fed calves
  - Other dairy stock (bulls, steers)

Feed supplies

- Enough fresh forage fed each day? Typical amount fed per milking cow in wet/dry season
- State of forage (improved v native v forage by-products, immature v mature)
- Sourcing fresh forage, grown v off farm
- Enough concentrates fed each day? Typical amount fed per cow
- Concentrates (formulated v mixed)
- What by-products are fed
- If on farm mixing, specific feed additives (macro minerals, vitamins/minerals, rumen buffers)
- Use of shed effluent for forage production

Answers to simple questions

- How many cows did you milk yesterday?
- How much milk did you sell yesterday?
- How much milk did you use to feed your milk-fed calves yesterday?

These answers should allow you to calculate the average milk yield per milking cow

- How much per litre of milk were you paid yesterday?
- If there is a milk grading scheme, what grade was your milk yesterday?
- What was the typical composition of your milk (fat, solids not fat, protein)?
- What was the typical quality of your milk (somatic cell count, TPC or MBRT)?

Answers to more complex questions

- How aware are you of the importance of colostrum feeding to your newborn calves and what are your normal practices?
- Do you keep any farm records? If so, which ones?
- What financial/business records do you keep?
- Do you consider mastitis to be a problem?
- Do you consider cow lameness to be a problem?
- What is the typical peak yield of your cows in early lactation?
- What is the typical lactation length of your cows (< 250, 250–275, 275–300, > 300 days)?

- What are your typical number of days between calving to conception?
- What is your typical number of days between cows drying off and then calving?
- What is your typical age (number of months) of heifers when they first calve down?
- What is your typical percentage of calves that show signs of ill health during milk rearing?
- What is your typical percentage of calves that die during milk rearing?
- How many years have you been milking cows?
- Will you still be milking cows in 1 year's time or 5 years' time?
- Do your children want to follow you on the farm?
- Name three of your biggest problems on your farm. This can be any constraint at all, such as labour supplies, government/co-op or milk processor support and services, dry season forage supplies. Poor milk returns and high cost of production are universal problems for all small holder dairy farmers, so should not be included unless they are an obvious problem on this farm.

Appendix 3 Cow signals to assess health and welfare

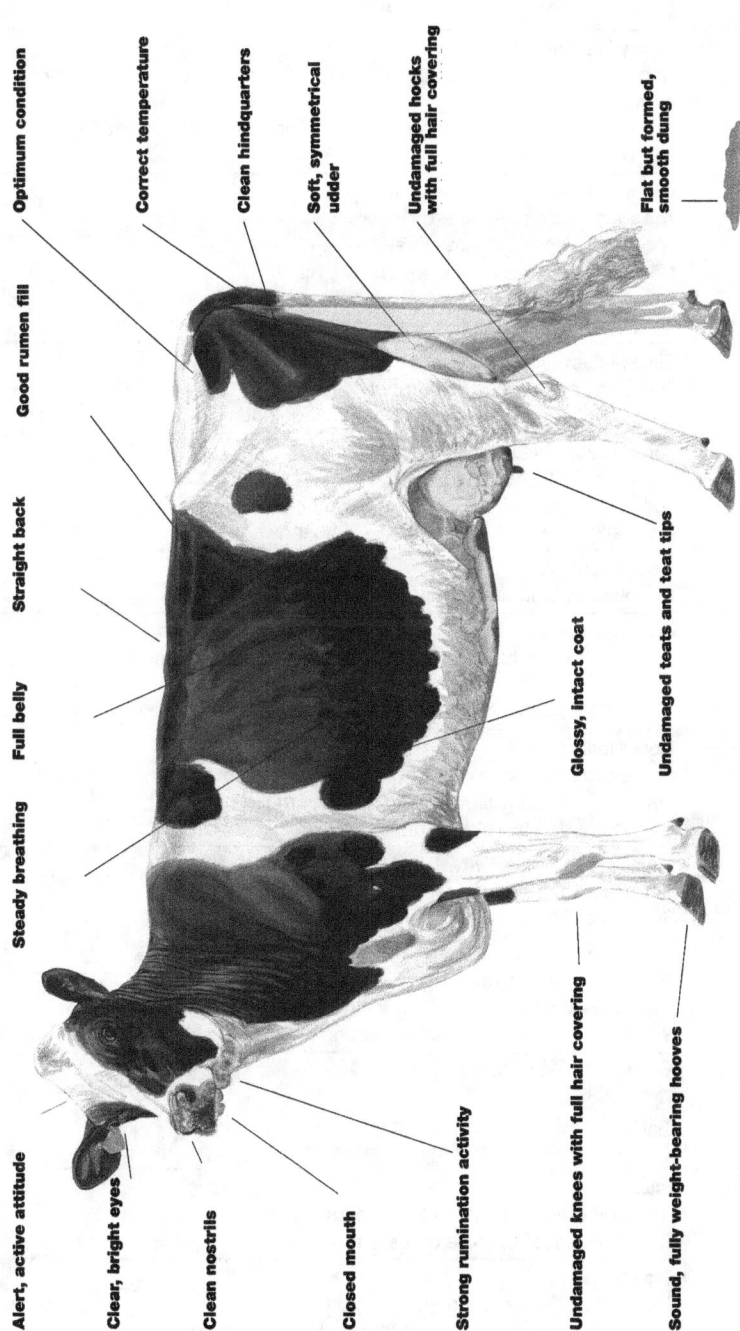

Alert, active attitude

Clear, bright eyes

Clean nostrils

Closed mouth

Strong rumination activity

Undamaged knees with full hair covering

Sound, fully weight-bearing hooves

Steady breathing

Full belly

Straight back

Good rumen fill

Glossy, intact coat

Undamaged teats and teat tips

Optimum condition

Correct temperature

Clean hindquarters

Soft, symmetrical udder

Undamaged hocks with full hair covering

Flat but formed, smooth dung

Cow's anatomy	Observation and interpretation
Whole body	**Alert, active attitude** Distracted attitude: poor health, low energy status and possibly rumen acidosis
	Steady breathing Rapid and shallow: heat stress or pain. Sometimes at start of rumination period as well Normal: 10 to 30 times per minute (in temperate regions), < 50 times per minute (in tropical regions)
	Optimum condition Too thin: inadequate energy intake Too fat: excessive energy intake Normal: good flesh cover with a little fat Good condition leads to improved disease resistance, fertility and health around calving (pay attention to breed)
	Glossy intact coat Dull coat: poor health or nutrition Skin injuries: cause and result of agitation and reduced disease resistance
	Correct body (rectal) temperature Too high (> 39.0°C): fever Too low (< 38.0°C): milk fever or serious illness Normal (between 38.0 and 38.5°C): healthy
Head	**Clear, bright eyes** Deep set eyes indicate cow is sick and dehydrated
	Clean nostrils Mucus with pus/blood and skin injuries: skin of the nose is inflamed due to virus or cold Clear mucus does not indicate much
	Closed mouth Some drooling: usually hunger Lot of drooling: swallowing problems or mouth pain Coughing: due to cold air, dust or disease
	Strong rumination activity Reduced chewing: diet lacks effective fibre Spitting out the cud: tooth problems, prickly bits in feed Normal: 55 to 75 chews per cud
Forequarters	**Undamaged knees with full hair covering** Bare knees: scraping on ground while getting up Swollen knees: bruising when getting up, lack of space in stall
	Sound, fully weight bearing hooves Tiptoeing, standing on tips of hooves Injured or swollen coronary band Eczema or scabs in interdigital space
Abdomen	**Full belly** Belly too empty: hadn't eaten enough last week Take account of the size of the calf, if any
	Good rumen fill Too empty: hasn't eaten enough yesterday No discernible layered structure (apple shaped): not enough fibre in diet

	Straight back Arched back: painful hooves or physical wear and tear Injuries: usually bruising against stall partition
Hindquarters	**Clean hindquarters** Dung on both sides of rump: dung too thin Asymmetric soiling: environment too dirty
	Soft, symmetrical udder Hard: due to oedema around calving or mastitis (painful) Enlarged quarter: active mastitis Shrunken quarter: previous mastitis
	Undamaged teats and teat tips Trodden teats: too much agitation, stalls too narrow or too slippery Check milking machine and technique if you see calloused teat tips: incorrect action of milking machine Swelling, redness or tiny blood spots: also due to udder oedema
	Undamaged hocks with full hair covering Bare hocks: scraping on stall floor, lack of grip Thick hocks: lack of stall space, stall floor too hard Scabs: inflammation due to dirt or moisture
	Flat but formed, smooth dung Long stems: insufficient rumination activity Not too loose or too firm: always relate to ration components (e.g. grazed pastures) and lactation stage (dry v peak lactation) Use dung feedback to assess the diet: feeding methods, feed intake, digestion, water intake and health Discus with nutritionist when dung does not seem optimal

Appendix 4 Cow signals to assess sickness and distress

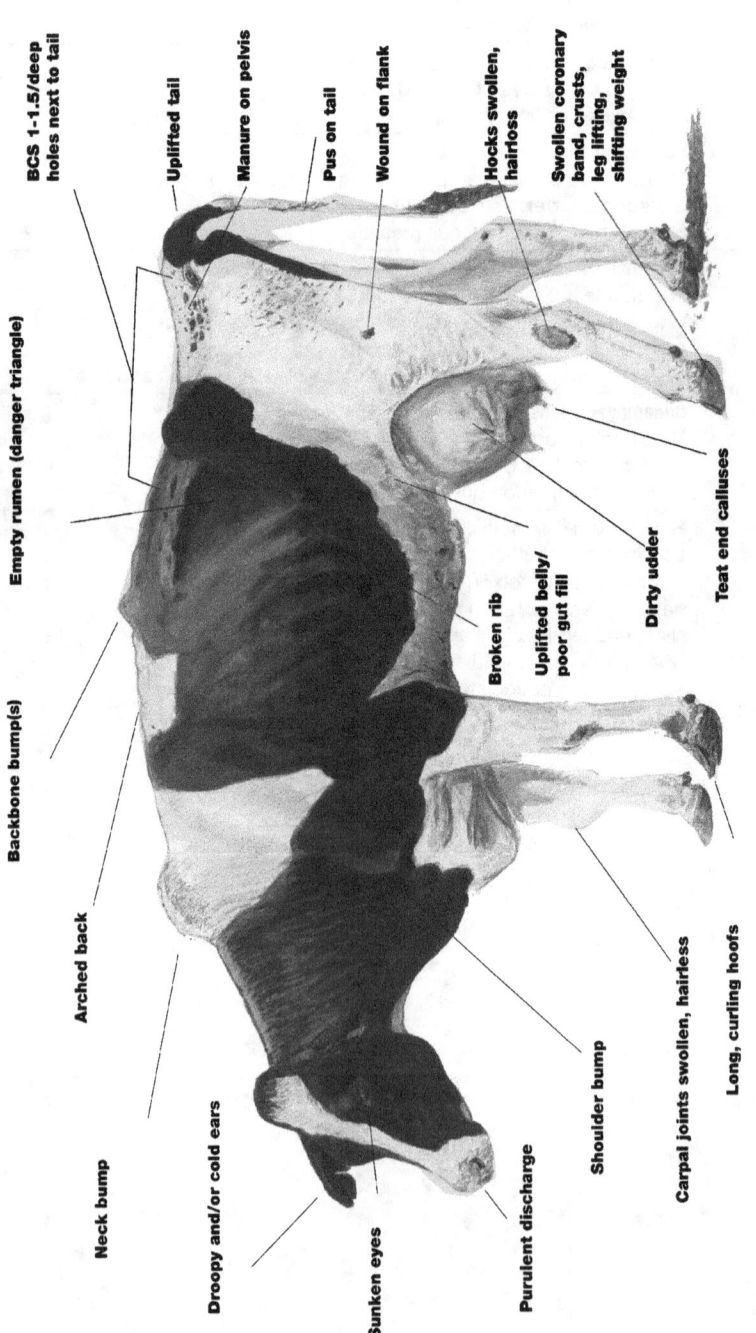

Cow's anatomy	Observation and interpretation
Head	Sunken eyes: sick
	Droopy and/or cold ears: sick
	Purulent nasal discharge: rhinitis or chronic lung problem
Forequarters	Neck bump: neck rail feed fence too low
	Shoulder bump: poorly designed feed fence/feed too far away
	Long curling hoofs: hoof trimming too late or not at all
	Carpal joints swollen, hairless: stall surface too hard, too little head space
Abdomen	Arched back: lame
	Backbone bumps: lying against stall divider
	Empty rumen: has eaten too little
	Broken rib: stall divider
	Uplifted belly/poor gut fill: pain/poor feed intake for days
Hindquarters	Body condition score of 1 to 1.5 and deep holes next to tail: long-term physical problems
	Dirty udder: dirty resting area and/or floors
	Teat end calluses: milking machine problems
	Uplifted tail: pain in birth canal
	Manure on pelvis: diarrhoea
	Pus on tail: endometritis
	Wound on flank: wet resting surfaces
	Swollen hocks and hair loss: stall surfaces too hard, abrasive or not enough grip
	Swollen coronary band, crusts, leg lifting, shifting weight: hoof diseases

Appendix 5   A scoring system to assess dairy cow welfare on any farm

This has been more fully described in Chapter 8 of this book. It contains 36 questions or observations. It is based on the 'five freedoms of animal welfare' and addresses both tethering and loose housing. As this scoring system was developed to focus more on good rather than poor animal welfare, the higher the scores, the better the welfare for the animals.

How to use this scoring system

1. Complete the details on farm. Animal numbers are important for score calculations.
2. Each of the 'five basic freedoms of animal welfare' is assessed.
3. Each measure is assigned a maximum value of 1.0. The total for each freedom is scored according to the number of measures answered. If the measure does not apply to that particular farm (for example it may not have any young calves), this should not be taken into account in the total.
4. For each measure, when 'yes' applies to more than 90% of animals, score 1.0 point. When 'yes' applies to 30% or less of animals, score 0.0 points. When 'yes' applies to 30–90% of animals, score 0.5 points.
5. Methods for scoring body condition, rumen fill, cleanliness, locomotion, hooves and teat scores are provided in Chapter 6 of this book.

Details of farm visited

Farm location	
Cooperative or feedlot	
Date and time of visit	
Owner/person responsible	
Total number of milking cows on farm	
Total number of calves on farm	

Summary of scores for each measure of animal welfare

Measure	Score
1. Freedom from hunger and thirst	
Do all animals (including calves) have continuous access to water?	
Are all feeders and drinkers functional?	
Are feeders and drinkers clean?	
Are cows in a body condition score between 2 and 4 out of 5 (Chapter 6.1)?	
Do cows have a rumen score appropriate to their point of calving (Chapter 6.6)?	
Are calves fed colostrum?	
Are cows fed a quality mixed ration?	
TOTAL	

2. Freedom from discomfort	
Do cows have a cleanliness score of 2 or less out of 5 (Chapter 6.5)?	
Is bedding provided?	
Is bedding clean and deep enough for cows to lie comfortably?	
Can animals lie down and get up easily?	
Is there shelter from extreme weather?	
Are cows free from hock sores?	
Are cows free from pressure sores?	
Are cows free from any signs of heat stress (< 70 breaths per minute)?	
TOTAL	
3. Freedom from pain, injury and disease	
Are cows free from injuries on their bodies?	
Do cows have a locomotion score of 2 or less out of 5 (Chapter 6.2)?	
Are cows free from clinical disease?	
Do cows have healthy hooves (e.g. no incidences of diseases described in Chapter 6.3)?	
Do cows have clean, healthy looking udders?	
Do cows have teat scores of 2 or less out of 4 (Chapter 6.8)?	
Do cows have their tails intact?	
Have calves been disbudded (not dehorned)?	
Have any male calves been castrated at 3 months of age or less?	
TOTAL	
4. Freedom from fear and distress	
Do cows approach the stockperson?	
Do calves approach the stockperson?	
Will the cows let the stockperson approach within 3 m?	
Can cows be moved gently, without hitting, yelling?	
Will cows walk slowly, not run, when encouraged to move by the stockperson?	
TOTAL	
5. Freedom to express normal behaviour	
Are cows free to move (untethered)?	
If tethered, are cows given access to move freely each day?	
Are calves housed in appropriate groups (between 2 and 8)?	
Can animals turn around fully in their cubicle?	
Is there a minimum of dry lying area of 3.5 m² for adult cattle/bulls and 2.5 m² for growing heifers?	
Is there evidence of normal social behaviours (limited aggressive interactions during feeding and resting)?	
Are stereotypical behaviours minimal?	
TOTAL	

The framework to calculate the animal welfare status of each farm visited is presented below. It is based on calculating a single value for each of the five freedoms then developing an animal welfare index based on equal weightings to each of these five freedoms.

Calculation of an animal welfare index for the farm visited

1. Freedom from hunger and thirst	
Total number of measures recorded (A); maximum of 7	
Sum of scores recorded (B)	
% score for Measure 1 (A/B x 100)	
2. Freedom from discomfort	
Total number of measures recorded (A); maximum of 8	
Sum of scores recorded (B)	
% score for Measure 2 (A/B x 100)	
3. Freedom from pain, injury and disease	
Total number of measures recorded (A); maximum, of 9	
Sum of scores recorded (B)	
% score for Measure 3 (A/B x 100)	
4. Freedom from fear and distress	
Total number of measures recorded (A); maximum of 5	
Sum of scores recorded (B)	
% score for Measure 4 (A/B x 100)	
5. Freedom to express normal behaviour	
Total number of measures recorded (A); maximum of 7	
Sum of scores recorded (B)	
% score for Measure5 (A/B x 100)	
6. Farm animal welfare index	
Mean value of all five % above	

Appendix 6   Animal welfare agencies in Australia

Shown below are the non-government and government agencies in Australia actively involved in animal welfare activities, including cattle.

Non-government organisations

Royal Society for the Protection of Cruelty to Animals (RSPCA)
    http://www.rspca.org.au/
Animals Australia
    http://www.animalsaustralia.org/
World Animal Protection
    http://www.worldanimalprotection.org
Voiceless
    https://www.voiceless.org.au/
People for Ethical Treatment of Animals (PETA)
    http://www.peta.org/
Australian Veterinary Association
    http://www.ava.com.au/

Government agencies

Australian Livestock Export Corporation (MLA/LIVECORP)
    http://www.livecorp.com.au/animal-welfare
Department of Agriculture, Fisheries and Forestry, Animal and Plant Health, Canberra
    http://www.daff.gov.au/animal-plant-health/welfare
Animal Welfare Science Centre, University of Melbourne, Victoria and Victorian Department of Environment and Primary Industries, Melbourne
    http://www.animalwelfare.net.au/
State governments
    Many state government agriculture departments employ animal welfare specialists
Universities
    Many of the veterinary science faculties at universities employ animal welfare specialists.
The World Association for Animal Health (OIE) is one of the key international agencies responsible for animal welfare with headquarters in Paris and website http://www.oie.int/animal-welfare/animal-welfare-key-themes/

Glossary

acidosis (or grain poisoning) This occurs when rumen pH falls too low through overproduction of lactic acid (the end product of grain digestion) which reduces feed digestion and sometimes causes death.

ad lib* or *ad libitum Fed to appetite (freely available to the cow).

age at first calving (AFC) A good indicator of heifer management in year-round calving herds. In seasonal-calving herds it is usually predetermined at about 24 months of age.

agonistic behaviour A form of social interaction that is associated with aggression, and that also includes threatening and submissive behaviour.

baulking Occurs when an animal flinches and ceases movement, often in response to something unfamiliar.

bar biting This is a stereotype behaviour when stock clamp their jaws around a bar of their stall and move their head back and forth while chewing on the bar for a minute or more.

best management practice (BMP) A description of the most suitable procedures for undertaking a set of tasks to develop a checklist for planning various activities on the farm. Basically it is 'saying what you do, doing what you say, then recording what you have done'.

biosecurity A strategy of management practices to prevent introduction of disease and pathogens to the operation and to control spread within the operation.

blind spot The area behind the cow which she cannot see. Sudden movement in this area will cause her to startle.

body condition A subjective estimate of the amount of subcutaneous fat between the pin bones and the tail head, over the hip and covering the lumbar vertebrae.

calving interval The average time period between consecutive calvings in a dairy herd. The target is 12 months, although this is rarely achieved.

cattle talkers Lengths of leather strips attached to cane to encourage cattle to move along the laneways; also known as 'cattle flappers'.

claw One of the two digits of a cow's foot.

close-up group Non-lactating pregnant milking cows due to calve within 3 weeks.

comfort zone The range of air temperature when there is no measurable fluctuation in physiological processes of cattle.

colostrum The milk produced by cows for the first two milkings post-calving which contains high levels of nutrients and immunoglobulins for transferring immunity into newborn calves.

conception rate The proportion of the total number of services or inseminations that result in pregnancy.

conception to calving interval The time period between when a cow has a calf and she next becomes pregnant.

contract heifer rearing The term used when dairy producers develop formal agreements with other graziers to grow out their heifers, usually at a predetermined growth rate, until point of calving.

cope To have control of mental and bodily stability or maintain control of mental and bodily stability in the face of a challenge.

cowpersonship The term could be defined as knowing the individual behaviour of every animal in one's charge and having the ability to recognise small changes in the behaviour of any animal or all the animals collectively.

cow trainers These are electric wires located above free and tie stalls to train cows not to contaminate their stalls with faeces and urine.

crude protein A crude measure of the total protein in a feed, calculated as the total nitrogen content multiplied by 6.25. It includes true protein, which provides the amino acids for animal use, and also non-protein nitrogen, such as urea.

cubicle A place for a single cow to stand or lie, which is separated from other cubicles by walls or dividers. The cows are not tied in the cubicle and can enter and leave at will. It is also called a stall.

dry matter (DM) The proportion of a feed remaining after being dried at 80 to 100°C for 24 hours or until a constant dry weight is achieved. The nutritive value and the livestock requirements of feeds are usually expressed on a dry matter, rather than a fresh weight basis.

E. coli Bacteria causing scours in calves.

euthanise Slaughter of animal because of health issue rather than because it has reached its planned slaughter live weight.

farm blindness Thinking that what you see every day around the farm is normal.

far-off group Pregnant milking cows that have just been dried off and are at least 3 weeks from calving.

fibre The cell wall, or structural material, in a plant made up of (among other things) cellulose, hemicellulose, and lignin.

fitness describes physical welfare, e.g. freedom from disease, injury and incapacity.

flehman response This is found in mating bulls (and cows mating other cows on heat) where the head is directed upwards with the mouth ajar, the tongue flat and the upper lips curled back.

flight distance or zone The 'personal' space around animals where they will attempt to move away from people.

foul-in-the-foot A term used to describe a disease syndrome in cows' feet resulting from wet feet and dirty floors.

grooming The cleaning of the body surface or rearrangement of hair on the coat by licking, nibbling, picking, rubbing or scratching. Grooming may be performed by the animal itself or by a social companion.

hierarchy An ordered sequence of individuals or groups of individuals in a social system which is based upon some ability or characteristic, most often to act aggressively towards or displace group members or to have priority of access to some areas of the cowshed.

indicator animals These belong to certain groups of stock on the farm that are at greater risk than others, so they are often the first to send out signals indicating something is wrong.

indicator (risk) locations These are risk locations on the farm where stock are more likely to be injured, such as a long rough track where small stones can injure hooves, or the calf shed where sudden changes in weather can upset calf wellbeing.

Key Performance Indicator (KPI) A numerical descriptor of some aspect of herd management or farm performance that can be used as a realistic target for future improved farm management programs.

lactation anoestrus This occurs when high genetic merit cows utilise excess levels of their body reserves to maintain milk yields. This means they will rapidly lose weight and upset the hormonal balances that allow them to regain their normal oestrus cycle soon after calving.

metabolisable energy (ME) The amount of energy provided by a feed after deducting energy lost to faeces,

urine, heat, and gas production; it is the energy available to be used by the animal for its metabolic activities.

MJ ME/kg DM Megajoules of metabolisable energy per kilogram of dry matter.

OIE The abbreviation for the French version of World Association for Animal Health which is one of the key international agencies responsible for animal welfare.

pH A measure of acidity or alkalinity on a scale from 1 (extremely acid) to 14 (extremely alkaline).

pheromone Chemicals produced by cows to indicate particular emotions, such as fear or being ready for mating, which trigger specific behavioural responses.

point of balance The position within the flight zone of the cow (near the shoulder) where she will either move forwards or backwards depending on the cow handler's movements.

quality In relation to feeds, it is an indication of the level of energy and digestibility. In relation to milk, it refers to the level of various contaminants in milk, such as bacterial, chemical or any other adulterations that can be detected.

quality assurance (QA) A structured set of best management practices.

risk locations These are locations on the farm where stock are more likely to be injured.

SE South-east.

service providers The farmer's network of people who provide services, equipment and 'good ideas' to improve their farm performance, profits and hence long-term sustainability.

SHD   Small holder dairy.

slatted floor   A combination of solid parts (slats), which would support the lower surface of the claw of the cow, and gaps (slots) which would allow manure and other liquids to pass through (also called slotted floor).

solid floor   A continuous flat surface which might be made of various materials and which allows full contact with and support to the lower surface of the claw of the cow.

social dominance groups   Herd have a clear social hierarchy which is made up of groups of cows with a similar social status within the herd.

Standard Operating Procedures (SOP)   A set of instructions for any activity or set of tasks undertaken on the farm.

stereotype behaviour   Repeated sequences of a behaviour that has no apparent purpose or benefit and is caused by the frustration of natural behaviour patterns or repeated attempts to deal with some problem. Tongue rolling and bar biting are two such examples in intensively housed cattle.

stress   An environmental effect on an individual that overtaxes its control systems and reduces its performance and survivability or has the potential to do so.

supplement   A feed or product added to the animal's diet to increase the intake of some dietary component, such as energy, protein, fibre, vitamins or minerals.

Temperature Humidity Index (THI)   A system for quantifying heat stress based on temperature and humidity. The higher the index, the greater the discomfort, and this occurs at lower temperatures for higher humidities.

thermoneutral zone   The temperature range within which metabolic heat production and energy expenditure are minimal, most productive processes are at their most efficient level and an animal is thermally comfortable without the need to change heat production. The zone is limited by the lower critical temperature (LCT) and the upper critical temperature (UCT); above and below there are energy costs of thermoregulation.

tongue rolling   This is a stereotype behaviour in which animals extrude and move their tongue by curling and uncurling it inside or outside their mouth. After that, partial swallowing of the tongue and gulping of the air can take place.

unclassified notable observations (UNO)   (or 'you know') Observations of cow behaviour or cow signals that do not always have a logical explanation. At first glance, these may appear to be insignificant, but on reflection and further consideration, they can become important.

vomeronasal organ   This is a smell (olfactory) sensitive organ located in cattle on the roof of their mouth. The reception of odours by this organ is used for the reinforcement and maintenance of sexual interest.

wastage rate   A measure of losses in replacement heifers between birth and second calving.

water lapping   This occurs when some cows lick the water with their tongue instead of putting their mouth in contact with the water and syphoning it into their mouth.

white line disease   A term used to describe a disease condition of cows' feet where there is a break in the continuity between the white (or pink) line and the wall of the sole.

withholding period   The number of days following drug administration before milk or meat can be sold from treated animals.

zoonoses   Cattle diseases that can be passed onto humans.

Abbreviations

Other less common abbreviations are included in the glossary.

A	Australian	m	metre
AI	artificial insemination	mg	milligram
C	Centigrade	MJ	megajoule
c	cents	min	minute
Ca	calcium	mm	millimetre
cm	centimetre	mth	month
d	day	N	nitrogen
F	Fahrenheit	P	phosphorus
g	gram	pa	per annum
ha	hectare	s	seconds
hd	head	SE	South-East (Asia)
h	hour	T	tonnes
Hz	hertz (a measure of sound frequency)	US	United States of America
		yr	year
kg	kilogram	<	less than
L	litre	>	greater than
LWT	live weight	$	dollar
lux	lux (a measure of light intensity)		

References and further reading

Albright JL, Arave CW (1997) *The Behaviour of Cattle*. CAB International, Oxford, UK.

Albright JL, Fulwider WK (2007) Dairy cattle behaviour, facilities, handling, transport, automation and well-being. In *Livestock Handling and Transport*. 3rd edn. (Ed. T Grandin) pp. 109–133. CAB International, Oxford, UK.

AssureWel (2010) *Advancing Animal Welfare Assurance*. Collaborative project of University of Bristol, RSPCA and Soil Association of UK. <http://www.assurewel.org/dairycows>

Blaszak K (2011) *WSPA report: dairy cattle industry and welfare in Indonesia*. World Society for Protection of Animals, Sydney, Australia.

Bos AP, Cornelissen JMR, Koerkamp PWG (2009) *Cow Power: Designs for System Innovation*. Wageningen, Lelystad, Netherlands.

Brambell FWR (1965) *Report of the technical committee to enquire into the welfare of animals kept under intensive livestock husbandry systems*. Command paper 2836, HMSO London, UK.

Chenoweth PJ, Landaeta-Hernandez AJ (1998) Maternal and reproductive behaviour of livestock. In *Genetics and the Behaviour of Domestic Animals*. (Ed. T Grandin) pp. 145–165. Academic Press, Elsevier, US.

Delgardo C, Rosegrant M, Wada N (2003) Meating and milking global demand: stakes for small-scale farmers in developing countries. In *The Livestock Revolution: A Pathway to Poverty?* pp. 13–23. ATSE Crawford Fund Conference, Canberra, Australia.

European Food Safety Authority (2009) Scientific opinion on the overall effects of farming systems on dairy cow welfare and disease. *The EFSA Journal* **1143**, 1–38.

FAOSTAT (2010) FAO statistics online. <http://faostat3.fao.org/faostat-gateway/go/to/browse/Q/QP/E>

Farm Animal Welfare Council (2009) *Five Freedoms*. <http://www.fawc.org.uk/freedoms.htm>

Food and Agriculture Organisation (2011) *Guide to good dairy farming practice*. Animal health and production guidelines no 8. FAO and IDF, Rome, Italy.

Fraser D, Weary DM, Pajor EA, Milligan BN (1997) A scientific conception of animal welfare that reflects ethical concerns. *Animal Welfare (South Mimms, England)* **6**, 197–205.

Grandin T (Ed.) (1998) *Genetics and the Behaviour of Domestic Animals*. Academic Press, Elsevier, US.

Grandin T (Ed.) (2007) *Livestock Handling and Transport*. 3rd edn. CAB International, Oxford, UK.

Grandin T, Deesing MJ (1998) Genetics and animal welfare. In *Genetics and* the *Behaviour of Domestic Animals.* (Ed. T Grandin) pp. 319–346. Academic Press, Elsevier, US.

Graves RE, McFarland F, Tyson JT (2009) *Designing and Building Dairy Cattle Free Stalls.* PennState College of Agricultural Sciences, Pennsylvania, US.

Hemme T, Otto J (2010) *Status and prospects for smallholder milk production: a global perspective.* FAO, Rome.

Hemsworth PH, Coleman GJ, Barnett JL, Borg S, Dowling S (2002) The effects of cognitive behavioral intervention on the attitude and behavior of stockpersons and the behavior and productivity of commercial dairy cows. *Journal of Animal Science* **80**, 68–78.

Hooten N (2008) Dairy development for the resource poor. Lessons for policy and planning strategies. In *Developing an Asian regional strategy for sustainable small holder dairy development.* pp. 48–51. Proceedings of an FAO/APHCA/CFC funded workshop, Chiang Mai, Feb 2008.

Hulsen J (2011) *Cow Signals: A Practical Guide for Dairy Farm Management.* Roodbont Publishers, Zutphen, Netherlands.

Hulsen J (2013) *Cow Signals Checkbook: Working on Health, Production and Welfare.* Roodbont Publishers, Zutphen, Netherlands.

International Dairy Federation (2008) *Guide to Good Animal Welfare in Dairy Production.* Brussels, Belgium.

Keidane I (2007) Research of physical and chemical environmental factors and their influence upon cows kept at cold cow-houses. In *Animal Health, Animal Welfare and Biosecurity.* Volume 1. (Ed. A. Aland) pp. 461–465. Proceedings of the 13th International Congress on Animal Hygiene, Tartu, Estonia, 2007.

Klindworth D, Greenall R, Campbell J (2003) *Cowtime guideline for milk harvesting.* Dairy Research and Development Corporation, Melbourne, Australia.

Mason G, Rushen J (2006) *Stereotypic Animal Behaviour: Fundamentals and Applications to Welfare.* 2nd edn. CABI, Oxfordshire, UK.

Meat and Livestock Australia or MLA (2006) *Recognising excessive heat load in feedlot cattle: tips and tools.* Meat and Livestock Australia, Sydney.

Milk Vita (2013) *Developmental activities at Milk Vita's Baghabari ghat dairy plant, Sirajgonj, Bangladesh.* Milk Vita, Sirajgonj, Bangladesh.

Moberg GP (2001) Biological response to stress: implications for animal welfare. In *The Biology of Animal Stress.* (Eds GP Moberg, JA Mench). CAB International, Wallingford, Oxon, UK.

Moran JB (2005) *Tropical Dairy Farming: Feeding Management for Small Holder Dairy Farms in the Humid Tropics.* CSIRO Publishing, Melbourne. <http://www.publish.csiro.au/nid/197/issue/3363.htm>

Moran JB (2009a) *Business Management for Tropical Dairy Farmers.* CSIRO Publishing, Melbourne. <http://www.publish.csiro.au/nid/220/issue/5522.htm>

Moran J (2009b) Key performance indicators to diagnose poor farm performance and profitability of smallholder dairy farmers in Asia. *Asian-Australasian Journal of Animal Sciences* **22**, 1709–1717.

Moran J (2011) Factors affecting high mortality rates of dairy replacement calves and heifers in the tropics and strategies for their reduction. *Asian-Australasian Journal of Animal Sciences* **24**, 1318–1328.

Moran JB (2012a) *Managing High Grade Dairy Cows in the Tropics.* CSIRO Publishing, Melbourne. <http://www.publish.csiro.au/nid/220/issue/6812.htm>

Moran JB (2012b) *Rearing Young Stock on Tropical Dairy Farms in Asia.* CSIRO Publishing, Melbourne. <http://www.publish.csiro.au/nid/220/issue/6810.htm>

Moran J (2013) Addressing the key constraints to increasing milk production from small holder dairy farms in tropical Asia. *International Journal of Agricultural Biosciences* **2**(3), 90–98.

Moran J (2014) *The feeding of by-products on small holder dairy farms in Asia and other tropical regions.* Final report of E-Conference held in November–December 2013. Asia Dairy Network. <www.dairyasia.org>

Moran J, Brouwer J (2013) Interrelationships between measures of cow and herd performance and farm profitability on Malaysian dairy farms. *International Journal of Agricultural Biosciences* **2**(5), 221–233.

Moran JB, Wood JT (1986) Comparative performance of five genotypes of Indonesian large ruminants. 3. Growth and development of carcass tissues. *Australian Journal of Agricultural Research* **37**, 435–447.

Nguhiu-Mwangi J, Aleri JW, Mogoa EGM, Mbithi PMF (2013) Indicators of poor welfare in dairy cows within smallholder zero grazing units in the peri-urban areas of Nairobi, Kenya. In *Insights from Veterinary Medicine.* (Ed. R Payan-Carreira) pp. 49–88. InTech Publishers, Rijeka, Croatia.

Office International des Epizooties (2013) *Terrestrial Animal Health Code.* World Organisation for Animal Health, Paris, France.

Phillips C (2002) *Cattle Behaviour and Welfare.* 2nd edn. Blackwell Publishing, Oxford, UK.

Price EO (1998) Behavioural genetics and the process of animal domestication. In *Genetics and the Behaviour of Domestic Animals.* (Ed. T Grandin) pp. 31–65. Academic Press, Elsevier, US.

Schreiner DA, Ruegg PL (2002) Effects of tail docking on milk quality and cow cleanliness. *Journal of Dairy Science* **85**, 2503–2511.

Sprechter DJ, Holstetler DE, Kaneene JB (1997) A lameness scoring system that uses posture and gait to predict dairy cattle reproductive performance. *Theriogenology* **47**, 1178–1187.

Stafford KJ, Mellor DJ (2005a) Dehorning and disbudding distress and its alleviation in calves. *Veterinary Journal (London, England)* **169**, 337–349.

Stafford KJ, Mellor DJ (2005b) The welfare significance of the castration of cattle: a review. *New Zealand Veterinary Journal* **53**, 271–278.

Svensson C, Lundborg K, Emanuelson U, Olsson S (2003) Morbidity in Swedish dairy calves from birth to 90 days of age and individual calf-level risk factors for infectious diseases. *Preventive Veterinary Medicine* **58**, 179–197.

Vasseur E, Pellerin D, de Passill AM, Winckler C, Lensink BJ, Knierim U, Rushen J (2012) Assessing the welfare of dairy calves: outcome-based measures of calf health versus input-based measures of the use of risky management practices. *Animal Welfare (South Mimms, England)* **21**, 77–86.

von Keyserlingk MAG, Rushen J, de Passille AM, Weary DM (2009) Invited review: the welfare of dairy cattle – key concepts and the role of science. *Journal of Dairy Science* **92**, 4101–4111.

Welfare Quality (2009) *Welfare quality assessment protocol for cattle*. Welfare Quality Consortium, Lelystad, Netherlands.

Whay HR, Main DCJ, Green LE, Webster AJF (2003) Assessment of the welfare of dairy cattle using animal-based measurements: direct observations and investigations of farm records. *The Veterinary Record* **153**(7), 197–202.

Zurbrigg K, Kelton D, Anderson N, Millman S (2005) Tie stall design and its relationship to lameness, injury and cleanliness on 317 Ontario dairy farms. *Journal of Dairy Science* **88**, 3201–3210.

Index

www.ingramcontent.com/pod-product-compliance
Lightning Source LLC
Chambersburg PA
CBHW081437170526
45166CB00008B/2230